Milestones in Drug Therapy
MDT

Series Editors

Prof. Dr. Michael J. Parnham
PLIVA
Research Institute
Prilaz baruna Filipovica 25
10000 Zagreb
Croatia

Prof. Dr. J. Bruinvels
INFARM
Sweelincklaan 75
NL-3723 JC Bilthoven
The Netherlands

Glucocorticoids

Edited by N.J. Goulding and R.J. Flower

Birkhäuser Verlag
Basel . Boston . Berlin

Editors

Nicolas J. Goulding
Dept of Biochemical Pharmacology
William Harvey Research Institute
Barts and the London School of Medicine
and Dentistry
Queen Mary, University of London
Charterhouse Square
London EC1M 6BQ
UK

Rod J. Flower
Dept of Biochemical Pharmacology
William Harvey Research Institute
Barts and the London School of Medicine
and Dentistry
Queen Mary, University of London
Charterhouse Square
London EC1M 6BQ
UK

Library of Congress Cataloging-in-Publication Data

Glucocorticoids / ed. by N.J. Goulding and R.J. Flower.
    p. ; cm. – (Milestones in drug therapy)
    Includes bibliographical references and index.
    ISBN 3764360593 (alk. paper)
    1. Glucocorticoids–Therapeutic use, I. Goulding, N. J. (Nicolas J.), 1956- II. Flower,
R. J. (Rod J.), 1945- III. Series.
    [DNLM: 1. Glucocorticoids–pharmacolgy. 2. Glucocorticoids–physiology. 3.
Glucocorticoids–therapeutic use. WK 755 G5675 2001]
    RM292.3 G58 2001
    615'.364–dc21   00-066774

Deutsche Bibliothek Cataloging-in-Publication Data

Glucocorticoids / ed. by N. J. Goulding and R. J. Flower. - Basel ; Boston ; Berlin : Birkhäuser, 2001
(Milestones in drug therapy)
ISBN 3-7643-6059-3

ISBN 3-7643-6059-3 Birkhäuser Verlag, Basel - Boston - Berlin

© 2001 Birkhäuser Verlag, P.O. Box 133, CH-4010 Basel, Switzerland
Birkhäuser is a member of the BertelsmannSpringer Publishing Group
Printed on acid-free paper produced from chlorine-free pulp. TFC ∞
Cover illustration: Schematic representation of the human glucocorticoid receptor (see p. 7)
Printed in Germany
ISBN 3-7643-6059-3
9 8 7 6 5 4 3 2 1

Contents

The development of glucocorticoids as therapeutic agents

Molecular mechanisms of glucocorticoid action

Current perspectives in glucocorticoid biology

List of contributors

Filip J. Baert, Department of Gastroenterology, University Hospital Gasthuisberg, Herestraat 49, 3000 Leuven, Belgium; e-mail: baert.delsupehe@village.uninet.be

Dimitrios T. Boumpas, National Institutes of Health, Bethesda, MD 20892-1828, USA, and Division of Rheumatology, Clinical Immunology and Allergy, University of Crete, Heraklion 71300, Greece; e-mail: boumpasd@med.voc.gr

Julia C. Buckingham, Department of Neuroendocrinology, Division of Neuroscience & Psychological Medicine, Imperial College School of Medicine, Charing Cross Hospital, Fulham Palace Road, London W6 8RF, UK; e-mail: j.buckingham@ic.ac.uk

John A. Cidlowski, Laboratory of Signal Transduction, National Institute of Environmental Health Sciences, P.O. Box 12233, MD E2-02, Research Triangle Park, North Carolina 27709, USA; e-mail: cidlowski@niehs.nih.gov

Anne-Marie Cowell, Department of Neuroendocrinology, Division of Neuroscience & Psychological Medicine, Imperial College School of Medicine, Charing Cross Hospital, Fulham Palace Road, London W6 8RF, UK; e-mail: anne-cowell@supanet.com

Jamie D. Croxtall, William Harvey Research Institute, St. Bartholomew's and the Royal London School of Medicine, University of London, Charterhouse Square, London EC1M 6BQ, UK; e-mail: J.Croxtall@qmw.ac.uk

Marc B. Feinstein, John Hopkins Asthma and Allergy Center, 5501 Hopkins Bayview Circle, Baltimore, MD 21224-6801, USA; e-mail: feinstein@mskc.org

John R. Kirwan, University Division of Medicine, Bristol Royal Infirmary, Bristol BS2 8HW, UK; e-mail: John.Kirwan@Bristol.ac.uk

Allan Munck, Department of Physiology, Dartmouth Medical School, Lebanon NH 03756-0001, USA; e-mail: Allan.U.Munck@Dartmouth.edu

Robert H. Oakley, Laboratory of Signal Transduction, National Institute of Environmental Health Sciences, P.O. Box 12233, MD E2-02, Research Triangle Park, North Carolina 27709, USA; e-mail: roakley@norakbio.com

Fotini Paliogianni, Department of Microbiology, University of Patra, Patra 26224, Greece

Luca Parente, Department of Pharmaceutical Sciences, University of Salerno, Via Ponte Don Melillo, 84084 Fisciano (Salerno), Italy; e-mail: lparente@unisa.it

Mauro Perretti, William Harvey Research Institute, St. Bartholomew's and the

Royal London School of Medicine, University of London, Charterhouse Square, London EC1M 6BQ, UK; e-mail: M.Peretti@qmw.ac.uk

Niccoló Pipitone, Rheumatology Unit, GKT School of Medicine, Guy's Campus, London SE1 9RT, UK

Costantino Pitzalis, Rheumatology Unit, GKT School of Medicine, Guy's Campus, London SE1 9RT, UK; e-mail: costantino.pitzalis@kd.ac.uk

Paul R. Rutgeerts, Department of Gastroenterology, University Hospital Gasthuisberg, Herestraat 49, 3000 Leuven, Belgium; e-mail: paul.rutgeerts@uz.kuleuven.ac.be

Robert P. Schleimer, John Hopkins Asthma and Allergy Center, 5501 Hopkins Bayview Circle, Baltimore, MD 21224-6801, USA; e-mail: rschleim@welch.jhu.edu

John H. Toogood, The London Health Sciences Centre, South Campus (Victoria), Allergy Clinic, 800 Commissioners Road, East, London, Ontario, Canada N6A 4G5, UK

Preface

When, in 1949, Hench and his colleagues of the Mayo Clinic presented their findings on the dramatic anti-inflammatory effects of cortisol and cortisone to the Seventh International Congress on Rheumatic Diseases, they introduced the world to a new type of therapeutic agent which found utility across the whole field of medicine. Indeed, as one reviewer [1] wittily remarked, "Therapy was now dated BC (before cortisone) or after (AC)!"

The story of the development of the glucocorticoids as drugs for the treatment of rheumatoid arthritis, skin disorders, asthma and many other conditions is of course, well known. But like their counterparts, the non-steroidal anti-inflammatory drugs, it was only many years after their discovery as therapeutically useful agents, that their mode of action was even partially elucidated.

Early investigators in this field took a physio-chemical view of this problem. However, the research changed direction, following the discovery of the intracellular receptor, and with the increasing awareness of the fact that many effects of these agents were mediated indirectly, through changes in gene expression.

Paradoxically, this new understanding also complicated further detailed investigation into their mechanism. To answer the question "How do glucocorticoids work in this disease?" is a much more complicated prospect than with most drugs because of the plethora of genes and proteins, whose expression are changed.

A researcher armed with the knowledge that approximately 1% of the genome may be regulated by glucocorticoids, may have problems formulating a clear hypothesis to test! From such studies however, a group of genes have emerged which are regulated by the glucocorticoids in ways that implicate them in their anti-inflammatory effect.

Ironically, now that we have had a quarter of a century of research into the genomic mechanisms, interest is once again focussing upon non-genomic pathways of glucocorticoiod action – rapid effects which require occupation of the glucocorticoid receptor, but not any genomic sequalae.

The purpose of this book is to bring together the thoughts of many of the leading researchers in the field and to provide an overview of glucocorticoid research as it stands at the end of the 20th Century. It is our hope that this will serve not only to instruct, but also to suggest future avenues for investigation and clinical application.

The glucocorticoid field has indeed become very large and to condense everything into a single volume would be very difficult. However, the contributors to the book have made valiant efforts to address most topics, including the basic biology of the glucocorticoids, and the development of the synthetic compounds which are mainly used for therapeutic purposes; there are extensive discussions to the glucocorticoid receptor, on the dynamics of cytokine and other gene regulation by these agents; the inter-relationship between exogenous and endogenous steroids and a discussion on the way in which the actions of endogenous steroids are regulated by the enzyme 11 beta hydroxy steroid dehydrogenase. Finally, there is a clinical section which deals with the use of steroids in asthma, arthritis and inflammatory bowel disease.

We would record our sincere thanks to all our contributors.

References

1 Hart FD (1983) Corticosteroid therapy in the rheumatic disorders. *In*: EC Huskisson (ed.) *Anti-rheumatic drugs*. Praeger, New York, 497–508

N.J. Goulding
R.J. Flower   October 2000

The development of glucocorticoids as therapeutic agents

Glucocorticoids
ed. by N.J. Goulding and R.J. Flower
© 2001 Birkhäuser Verlag/Switzerland

Glucocorticoid biology – a molecular maze and clinical challenge

Nicolas J. Goulding and Roderick J. Flower

Department of Biochemical Pharmacology, St Bartholomew's & the Royal London, School of Medicine & Dentistry, Queen Mary & Westfield College, London EC1M 6BQ, UK

Introduction

Over fifty years have now elapsed since glucocorticoids were first employed as anti-inflammatory drugs in the clinic. At that time, Dr Philip Hench and his colleagues at the Mayo Clinic made the seminal observation that administering an adrenal cortical steroid extract to a patient with progressive, active rheumatoid arthritis stopped the disease dead in its tracks [1]. This soon led to synthetic adrenal cortical steroids gaining a remarkable reputation in the treatment of a wide range of inflammatory and autoimmune disorders. However, it soon became apparent that this efficacy did not come without a cost in terms of potentially serious adverse effects. The fascinating history of glucocorticoid biology from Thomas Addison to the glucocorticoid receptor transgenic mouse is covered in the next chapter (A. Munck, this volume).

It is a poor reflection on the potency and specificity of currently available alternative anti-inflammatory therapy that glucocorticoids with all their caveats are still so widely employed today in the management of many diseases with autoimmune and inflammatory components. Admittedly, over the past five decades there has been an increasing degree of sophistication in their clinical application to try to minimise side-effects, but usage is still essentially empirical.

Glucocorticoids represent a classic therapeutic double-edged sword, with their profound anti-inflammatory activity balanced by serious risk of adverse effects in long-term, high dose use. Oral daily doses of >7.5 mg prednisolone or equivalent have been associated with increased incidence of osteoporosis and risk of fracture [2]. Doses of >20 mg prednisolone daily, significantly increase the risk of susceptibility to infection, HPA axis suppression as well as potential gastrointestinal, CNS, eye, muscle and cardiovascular problems. The development of synthetic glucocorticoids and an overview of these side-effects is given in the chapter of Parente. Even with these disadvantages, glucocorticoids remain pivotal agents in the management of a wide range of diseases with an autoimmune or inflammatory component. A recent study of the use of glucocorticoids in general practice estimated that over 250 000 patients in the UK are receiving continuous oral corticosteroid therapy [3].

A prime focus of clinical corticosteroid research is therefore to decrease the cost: benefit ratio of using these agents, and to a certain extent this is being achieved by increased sophistication in dosing schedules, routes of administration and the monitoring of side-effects. However, whilst the brunt of most current research is focused upon the pharmacological actions of high dose, high affinity synthetic steroids, it is clear that endogenous steroids also have important physiological activities in maintaining the body's "immune tone". It must not be forgotten that the natural human corticosteroid, cortisol, has mineralocorticoid as well as glucocorticoid activities and the 11β-hydroxysteroid dehydrogenase has a critical role in regulating the activity of endogenous glucocorticoids. (See chapter of Feinstein and Schleimer for a review of this field.) Likewise the body's response to inflammatory and immune stress in terms of HPA axis function and cortisol feedback is fundamental to resolution of inflammation (reviewed in the chapter of Cowell and Buckingham). Possible defects in this axis have been implicated in the development of chronic inflammatory disease. There is little doubt that these areas of research are ripe for future therapeutic exploitation.

Glucocorticoids and gene regulation

Glucocorticoids exert their manifold effects on cells involved in immune and inflammatory responses primarily by modulating the transcription of a large number of genes (it is estimated that they influence the transcription of approx-

Table 1. Corticosteroid effects on inflammatory mediators

Effect on transcription/translation	
Inhibition	Induction
Cytokines	
IL-1,-2,-3,-4,-5,-6,-11,-12,-13	IL-10, IL- 1RA
TNF-α, GM-CSF	
Chemokines	
IL-8, MCP-1,-3,-4	
RANTES, MIP-1α, eotaxin	
Adhesion molecules	
ICAM-1, E-selectin	
Receptors	
GR, NK$_1$, NK$_2$,	β2-adrenoceptor
IL-2R, IL-3R, IL-4R, IL-12R	IL-1R type I, IL-1R type II
	IL-6R
Enzymes and other mediators	
iNOS, COX-2, cPLA$_2$	Lipocortin 1 (annexin I)

imately 1% of the entire genome). However they are also able to influence the translational and post-translational mechanisms by which proteins are synthesised, processed and exported from cells. Table 1 illustrates the wide range of pro-inflammatory mediators whose production is influenced by glucocorticoids. These include cytokines, chemokines, enzymes and adhesion molecules. The majority of glucocorticosteroid effects are inhibitory but interestingly, glucocorticoids have been shown to increase the expression of several cytokine receptors including those for IL-1β and IL-6, which has led to a reexamination of the hypothesis of Hans Selye in the 1930s that at physiological concentrations, glucocorticoids can also have permissive effects on the immune system (see Munck, chapter 2). Volunteer studies in humans have also reported that glucocorticoids induce the production of endogenous anti-inflammatory proteins such as lipocortin 1 (AnxA1) [4], IL-10 [5], the IL1 receptor antagonist [6], and the IL1 type II "decoy" receptor [7]. The therapeutic potential of these proteins (along with many other currently uncharacterised glucocorticoid-induced proteins) may offer a degree of selectivity in corticosteroid mediated anti-inflammatory responses.

Multi-system effects of glucocorticoids

The clinical consequences of the widespread effects of glucocorticoids on many target cells, tissues and organs are well recognised and they stem from the fact that most cells in the body possess specific cytoplasmic and nuclear receptors for glucocorticoids known as glucocorticoid receptors (GR). The biology of the glucocorticoid receptor is extensively reviewed in the chapter of Oakley and Cidlowski. Thus, giving oral, systemic or intramuscular glucocorticoid therapy to a patient with rheumatoid arthritis will, in addition to the anticipated anti-inflammatory and immunomodulatory actions, also target glucose and lipid metabolism, the cardiovasculature, skeletal tissue, CNS and renal systems. These multi-system effects are summarised in Table 2. The clin-

Table 2. Effects of glucocorticoids on multiple organ systems and metabolic pathways

System	Effect
Cardiovasculature	Hypertensive – heightened pressor responses
Immune system	Immunosuppressive – leukocyte redistribution, maintenance of lymphoid tissues, feedback regulation of the HPA axis.
Kidney	Permissive action on tubular function and glomerular filtration
Skeleton	Maintenance of muscle tone and bone density
CNS	Regulation of neuronal excitability
Carbohydrate metabolism	Hyperglycaemia due to inhibition of insulin and stimulation of glucagon secretion
Lipid metabolism	Redistribution of body fat – increased lipolysis by adipocytes

ical benefit over risk ratio of a single bolus intravenous injection of methyl-prednisolone in an acute circumstance is usually acceptable as the short-term effects on these other systems are minimal compared to the profound effects on the immune system. However, long-term use of high dose corticosteroid therapy is accompanied by an increasing likelihood of adverse effects on these other physiological systems. Thus, future therapeutic strategies must move beyond a simple targeting of GR, with the key to greater specificity coming from emerging knowledge of the interaction of GR with DNA and other transcriptional regulators. This complexity is exemplified in the chapter of Paliogianni and Boumpas which deals with regulation of cytokine production by glucocorticoids.

Molecular mechanisms of action

Glucocorticoid receptors (see the chapter of Oakley and Cidlowski) are distributed in most human tissues with a common range of expression of the order of 3000–30 000 receptors per cell. GR are expressed in monocytes, macrophages, granulocytes and all lymphocyte sub-populations. Experimental adrenalectomy in rodents and the consequent fall in circulating endogenous corticosteroid results in increased GR expression by most tissues [8]. Conversely, GR levels fall in response to prolonged, elevated corticosteroid administration [9]. Modulation of GR expression may be associated with reduced cellular corticosteroid responsiveness. Recent studies have implied a link between the affinity of synthetic corticosteroid binding to GR in tissues and subsequent anti-inflammatory responsiveness [10].

The human GR was first isolated and cloned in 1985 [11]. Two alternate splice variants of a single gene have been described. The alpha form consists of 777 amino acids, the beta form of the receptor is expressed as a 742 amino acid protein, being truncated at the C terminus. The beta form of the receptor is unable to bind ligand although it has the capability to compete with the alpha form for DNA binding sites. The widespread expression of the beta form of the receptor in cells and tissues has led to speculation that it may function as an endogenous inhibitor of corticosteroid action but this remains controversial as mice totally lack such a receptor variant.

The ligand-binding GR protein is a molecule of 100 kDa and sequence data has confirmed it as a member of the nuclear steroid receptor superfamily which possess two characteristic "zinc-finger" motifs involved in DNA binding. Three functionally distinct areas of the GR molecule have been described. The major structure-function relationships are portrayed in Figure 1. The N-terminal region (τ 1) contains amino-acid sequences important for transactivation or transrepression of specific genes. The central "core" of the molecule is required for DNA binding, whilst the C-terminal domain contains the regions responsible for binding to the corticosteroid ligand and to a 90 kDa chaperone molecule which has been characterized as a heat shock protein (HSP 90) and whose

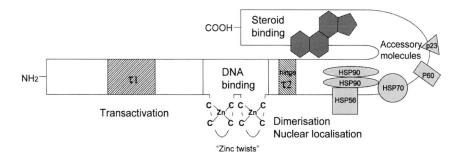

Figure 1. Schematic representation of the human glucocorticoid receptor showing functional regions and associated proteins.

probable function is to stabilise the receptor in the absence of ligand. Two HSP 90 molecules are associated with each GR and are released upon ligand binding, increasing the affinity of the receptor for DNA. Ligand binding also initiates receptor dimerisation which is important for the subsequent binding to DNA. Other regulatory molecules such as p23, p60, HSP56 and HSP60 are also involved in maintaining receptor structure and function.

Glucocorticoids are lipophilic molecules and so have the ability to pass easily through lipid membranes. Once inside the cytoplasm, subsequent actions have been classified according to their time-course of action and the dose required to produce the effect [12].

Genomic and non-genomic actions of glucocorticoids

GR-mediated events which mainly occur in the nucleus and involve interaction with DNA are classified as genomic whilst rapid effects which rely on other diverse interactions have been loosely termed non-genomic. The currently described modes of corticosteroid action are summarised in Table 3.

Genomic activities

The classical genomic action of glucocorticoids is relatively slow, occurring within hours, and is invoked by physiological concentrations of ligand. Figure 2 illustrates the sequence of events following binding of corticosteroid to the cytoplasmic GR. Ligand binding results in release of the HSP90 chaperone molecules and the ligand-receptor complex transmigrates to the nucleus (pathway a). Once within the nucleus, binding to specific sequences known as glucocorticoid response elements (GREs) within the promoter region of a particular gene results either in a downregulation (negative GRE) or upregulation (positive GRE) of its transcription. Following these effects, the receptor com-

Table 3. Diverse mechanisms of corticosteroid action

Action		Effect
Genomic		
Binding to GREs	- positive	Enhances transcription
	- negative	Inhibits transcription
	- composite (with other factors)	Variable
Interference with binding of other transcription factors		Variable
Non-genomic		
Reduction of mRNA stability		Inhibits translation
Intercollation in membranes		Reduces receptor activity
Binding to membrane receptors		Activates inhibitory signal transduction cascades
Prevention of DNA unwinding		Inhibits transcription
Condensation of chromatin structures		Inhibits transcription

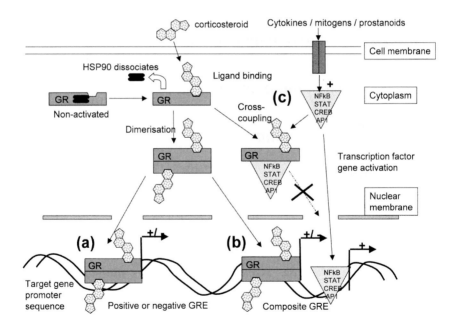

Figure 2. Identified genomic mechanisms of corticosteroid action. (a) Direct interaction of GR complex with DNA. (b) Binding to composite DNA elements with other transcription factors. (c) Interaction with other transcription factors remote from DNA which modulates genomic activity.

plex is released from DNA and recycled to the cytoplasm. These events occur within 1 h of corticosteroid administration as exemplified in Figure 3 which depicts GR staining in human peripheral blood mononuclear cells treated with

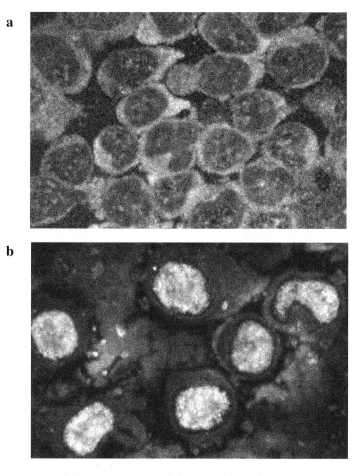

Figure 3. Expression of glucocorticoid receptor in human peripheral blood mononuclear cells cultured for 30 min (a) in the absence of corticosteroid (b) in the presence of 1×10^{-6} M dexamethasone. Confocal micrograph obtained using a Biorad MRC600 confocal microscope with 100 mW argon ion laser and 100× objective. The polyclonal anti-human GR was raised to a immunogenic peptide sequence in the N-terminal domain of both α and β forms of the receptor.

corticosteroid for 30 min. Added levels of complexity of corticosteroid action comes from the fact that activated GR has been shown to be able to interact with other transcription factors in the nucleus (Fig. 2, pathway b) which can influence its interaction with DNA at a promoter site know as a composite GRE and hence modulate gene transcription.

The gene regulatory regions of many inflammatory mediators inhibited by glucocorticoids do not contain GREs, which indicates that additional indirect mechanisms are very important. Strong evidence now exists that GR binding to DNA is not essential in order for corticosteroid to be effective. Whilst mice which have had the GR gene "knocked out" do not develop *in utero*, introduction of a mutation into the existing mouse GR gene which prevented its binding to GREs did not prevent the development and survival of engineered animals which appear healthy under normal laboratory conditions [13]. This and other evidence has led to the proposal that GR-ligand complexes can interfere with the activity of other transcription factors such as NF-κB and AP-1 without binding DNA (Fig. 2, pathway c).

One potential mechanism by which the activated GR complex may interfere with the transcription of a gene without involvement of direct DNA interaction has recently been identified. The interaction of a variety of intracellular transcription factors with a CREB-binding protein CBP is thought to be pivotal for the initiation of transcription mediated *via* the TATA-binding protein TBP. GR interaction with CBP/p300 inhibits binding of these factors and prevents activation of gene transcription [14, 15]. An increasing number of differentially expressed transcription factors are being identified which have the ability to interact with each other in this manner. The resulting effects on the transcription of pro-inflammatory genes indicates a fruitful, if complex, field of future research with the potential to "fine-tune" GR mediated effects on particular genes.

Non-genomic activities

Rapid effects of glucocorticoids occur which cannot be accommodated within the classical framework of interactions with DNA and transcription factors. These non-genomic actions of glucocorticoids have also been suggested as having important therapeutic implications, especially in the rheumatic diseases. Buttgereit and colleagues [16] have proposed a modular hypothesis for corticosteroid action. They suggest that endogenous glucocorticoids and low dose therapeutic steroids act through the classical pathways mediated by cytoplasmic GR. However, at prednisolone equivalents of $>1 \times 10^{-9}$ M, glucocorticoids can additionally act *via* cell surface GR [17]. By signaling through second messenger systems, these actions can occur in minutes rather than 1–2 h as is the case for genomic actions. However most of the evidence for such receptors comes from *in vitro* experiments in neuronal tissue and such actions on the immune system remain speculative, although they could explain the rapid negative feedback effect of glucocorticoids on ACTH production in the pituitary gland.

A second non-genomic action is suggested for very high doses of corticosteroid ($>1 \times 10^{-4}$ M prednisolone equivalent). Such doses can be achieved in patients receiving 1 g bolus intravenous doses of methylprednisolone. At these high doses, glucocorticoids are able to intercollate in biological membranes and exert physicochemical responses within a matter of seconds. This could potentially affect receptor motility and signaling as well as cationic membrane pumps and channels. Again, as with the intermediate module of surface receptor signaling, there is as yet no direct evidence that this mechanism can exert anti-inflammatory or immunosuppressive effects but the concept has provoked much debate.

In short, we are probably viewing the tip of a mechanistic iceberg as far as glucocorticoids are concerned. Reports of novel corticosteroid actions abound. One example is the ability of glucocorticoids to inhibit transcription of a large number of genes simultaneously by histone deacetylation, a process which prevents DNA unwinding, and promotes the formation of repressive chromatin structures [18].

Annexin 1 (AnxA1) – a mediator of glucocorticoid anti-inflammatory actions

Back in the late 1970s a protein termed "macrocortin" was isolated from macrophages which mediated several of the anti-inflammatory effects of glucocorticoids and whose transcription and translation appeared to be under the direct control of glucocorticoids [19]. DNA cloning and expression of the recombinant human protein led to its characterisation as a member of a family of calcium and phospholipid-binding proteins initially known as the lipocortins and now termed annexins (Anx). At least 200 members of this Anx family have now been characterised in mammals, lower animals, plants and protests. Each member of this multi-gene family possesses a characteristic highly homologous core region containing four 70 amino-acids subunits possessing a common sequence motif. Unique N-terminal domains appears to confer diverse physico-chemical characteristics and potential biological functions [20].

Annexin I is now classified as part of the AnxA mammalian protein classification, designated AnxA1. It has a molecular weight of 37 kDa and is found abundantly in mammalian tissues but has a discrete pattern of cellular distribution which includes secretory epithelium, skin, synovium and blood leukocytes [21]. A large body of evidence now exists to support the contention that synthesis of AnxA1 is controlled by glucocorticoids in these tissues and cells [22]. However, in certain transformed cell lines, expression of this protein appears to be associated with cell differentiation and growth rather than steroid concentration. The glucocorticoid regulation of AnxA1 is covered in the chapter of Croxtall whilst the chapter of Cowell and Buckingham reviews the role of AnxA1 in the early-delayed feedback loop of hypothalamo-pituitary adrenal (HPA) axis function.

A multitude of pharmacological studies in a wide range of animal models over the past 10 years have indicated a role for recombinant human lipocortin 1 (AnxA1) and derived peptides as potent inhibitors of inflammation, cytokine-mediated pyrogenesis and cerebral ischemia [23].

Evidence for an AnxA1 receptor

Extracellular actions of recombinant AnxA1 on cells involved in immune responses are significant and parallel some of the effects of glucocorticoids. Exogenous recombinant AnxA1 has been demonstrated to mimic corticosteroid suppression of monocyte functions such as superoxide generation [24] and autoimmune T lymphocyte profileration in response to myelin basic protein [25]. An indication that the exogenous protein may mediate its effects through specific cell surface receptors comes from the recent identification and characterisation of specific AnxA1 binding molecules on the surface of peripheral blood monocytes and polymorphonuclear leukocytes [26]. These binding sites are susceptible to proteolytic cleavage and are upregulated by only one cytokine, interleukin-10. The expression of these surface molecules on leukocytes from patients with rheumatoid arthritis is significantly reduced when compared to healthy individuals or patients with psoriasis or ankylosing spondilitis [27].

The existence of putative receptors for AnxA1 on human leukocytes and the lack of expression in a chronic inflammatory disease such as rheumatoid arthritis has led to the suggestion that it has a central role in glucocorticoid regulation of the inflammatory response [28].

Failure of this regulatory system may involve a defective HPA axis response to inflammatory or autoimmune injury (as reported in the Lewis rat [29]) resulting in reduced AnxA1 production, permitting chronic influx of activated leukocytes into the inflammatory site. Certainly AnxA1 production by peripheral blood leucocytes from patients with RA is impaired [30]. Furthermore, the presence of neutralising autoantibodies to AnxA1 which have been described in autoimmune diseases such as rheumatoid arthritis [31], systemic lupus erythematosus and in MRL autoimmune mice [32], or the deficiency in the expression of AnxA1 binding sites, as has recently been demonstrated in active rheumatoid arthritis [26], could be additional factors conspiring to perpetuate inflammatory and autoimmune activities and their pathological consequences.

AnxA1 and neutrophil transmigration

The migration of neutrophils from the peripheral circulation, through endothelial layers and into areas of tissue inflammation is critical to the host response to injury. Synovial exudates in rheumatoid arthritis are often characterised by the presence of large numbers of such cells. Much progress has been made over the last 10 years in our understanding of the mechanisms of neutrophil activation, and the expression of cell surface molecules involved in the adhesion of neutrophils to endothelial surfaces [33]. Less is known however about the process by which neutrophils extravasate into tissues and the mechanism by which this process stops when the inflammation is resolving. Glucocorticoids have a powerful negative effect on neutrophil extravasation and recent evidence suggests that AnxA1 may play an important role as a feedback control mechanism in this process (see the chapter of Pitzalis, Pipitone and Perretti for more detail on this).

Neutrophils have abundant intracellular stores of AnxA1 which have a granular localisation. Exposure of neutrophils to doses of corticosteroid similar to peak levels of endogenous steroid result in a rapid upregulation of AnxA1 within 2 h of administration [34]. Following adhesion of neutrophils to endothelium, this AnxA1 is mobilised and externalised [35]. Thus this externalisation of AnxA1 constitutes an endogenous autocrine negative feedback mechanism which regulates the inflammatory process by preventing further neutrophil accumulation. AnxA1 inactivation or sequestration could potentially fuel chronicity of neutrophil accumulation that is characteristic of the rheumatoid synovial exudate. (The chapter of Pitzalis, Pipitone and Perretti provides more detail on this mechanism.)

Future perspectives for glucocorticoid therapy

Whilst our current repertoires of synthetic glucocorticoids remain useful immunosuppressive and anti-inflammatory agents, there is plenty of scope for future improvements in their therapeutic use. The last three chapters summarise the use of glucocorticoids in asthma, arthritis and inflammatory bowel disease respectively and provide an indication of current good practice in these diseases. In the short-term future, better monitoring of corticosteroid efficacy based on biological responsiveness could reduce the risk of adverse effects by allowing dose-titering on an individual patient basis [36]. Also, development of "second-generation" glucocorticoids such as deflazacort, with reported "bone-sparing" properties, is also a promising trend, although the anti-inflammatory equipotency of this agent with prednisolone has been questioned [37].

So what about the long-term future? Advance in our understanding of the subtleties of the molecular interactions of endogenous corticosteroids with steroid receptors, transcription factors and DNA consensus sequences represents the first phase of this process. When this knowledge is interwoven with a greater understanding of the steroid regulation of anti-inflammatory mediators such as Annexin 1 and cytokines such as interleukin-10, novel research strategies will develop in three definable areas of research. Firstly in understanding how the immune system is homeostatically regulated, secondly in greater knowledge of the feedback resolution of the inflammatory response and finally and most crucially, in the development of new therapeutic modalities where beneficial anti-inflammatory or immunosuppressive effects can be dissected out from those unwanted effects on other tissues and organ systems.

References

1   Hench P, Kendall EC, Slocumb CH, Polley HF (1949) The effects of a hormone of the adrenal cor-
    tex and of pituitary adrenocorticotropic hormone on rheumatoid arthritis. *Proc Mayo Clin* 24:
    181–197
2   Eastell R, Reid DM, Compston J et al (1998) A UK Consensus Group on management of gluco-
    corticoid-induced osteoporosis: an update. *J Int Med* 244: 271–292
3   Walsh LJ, Wong CA, Pringle M, Tattersfield AE (1996) Use of oral glucocorticoids in the com-
    munity and the prevention of secondary osteoporosis: a cross sectional study. *Brit Med J* 313:
    344–346
4   Goulding NJ, Godolphin JL, Sharland PR et al (1990) Anti-inflammatory lipocortin 1 production
    by peripheral blood leucocytes in response to hydrocortisone. *Lancet* 335: 1416–1418
5   Tabardel Y, Duchateau J, Schmartz D et al (1996) Glucocorticoids increase blood interleukin-10
    levels during cardiopulmonary bypass in men. *Surgery* 119: 76–80
6   Levine SJ, Benfield T, Shelhamer JH (1996) Glucocorticoids induce intracellular interleukin-1
    receptor antagonist type I expression by a human airway epithelial cell line. *Amer J Respir Cell
    Mol Biol* 15: 245–251
7   Colotta F, Saccani S, Giri JG et al (1996) Regulated expression and release of the IL-1 decoy
    receptor in human mononuclear phagocytes. *J Immunol* 156: 2534–2541
8   Ovadia H, Sobcho A, Wholmann A, Weidenfeld J (1995) Cellular nuclear binding and retention of
    glucocorticoids   in   rat   lymphoid   cells: Effect   of   long-term   adrenalectomy.
    Neuroimmunomodulation 2: 339–346
9   Korn SH, Wouters EF, Wesseling G, Arends JW, Thunnissen FB (1997) *In vitro* and *in vivo* mod-
    ulation of alpha and beta glucocorticoid receptor mRNA in human bronchial epithelium. *Amer J
    Respir Crit Care Med* 155: 1117–1122
10 Hogger P, Rohdewald P (1998) Glucocorticoid receptors and fluticasone propionate. *Rev Contemp
    Pharmacotherapy* 9: 501–522
11 Hollenberg SM, Weinberger MC, Ong ES et al (1985) Primary structure and expression of a func-
    tional human glucocorticoid receptor cDNA. *Nature* 315: 635–641
12 Wehling M (1997) Specific, nongenomic actions of steroid hormones. *Annu Rev Physiol* 59:
    365–393
13 Reichardt HM, Kaestner KH, Tuckermann J et al (1998) DNA binding of the glucocorticoid recep-
    tor is not essential for survival. *Cell* 93: 531–541
14 Sheppard KA, Phelps KM, Williams AJ et al (1998) Nuclear intergration of glucocorticoid recep-
    tor and nuclear factor-kappa B signaling by CREB-binding protein and steroid receptor coactiva-
    tor-1. *J Biol Chem* 273: 29291–29294
15 Barnes PJ (1998) Anti-inflammatory actions of steroids: molecular mechanisms. *Clin Sci* 94:
    557–572
16 Buttgereit F, Wehling M, Burmester G-D (1998) A new hypothesis of modular glucocorticoid
    actions – Steroid treatment of the rheumatic diseases revisited. *Arthritis Rheum* 41: 761–767
17 Watson CS, Gametchu B (1999) Membrane-initiated steroid actions and the proteins that mediate
    them. *Proc Soc Exp Biol Med* 220: 9–19
18 Archer TK, Deroo BJ (1997) Chromatin modulation of glucocorticoid and progesterone receptor
    activity. *Trends Endocrinol Metab* 8: 384–390
19 Flower RJ (1984) Macrocortin and the antiphospholipase proteins. *Adv Inflam Res* 8: 1–34
20 Raynal P, Pollard HB (1994) Annexins: the problem of assessing the biological role for a gene
    family of multifunctional calcium- and phospholipid-binding proteins. *Biochim Biophys Acta*
    1197: 63–93
21 Fava RA, McKanna J, Cohen S (1989) Lipocortin I (p35) is abundant in a restricted number of
    differentiated cell types in adult organs. *J Cell Physiol* 141: 284–293
22 Vishwanath BS, Frey FJ, Bradbury M et al (1992) Adrenalectomy decreases lipocortin-I messen-
    ger ribonucleic acid and tissue protein content in rats. *Endocrinology* 130: 585–591
23 Flower RJ, Rothwell NJ (1994) Lipocortin-1: cellular mechanisms and clinical relevance. *Trends
    Pharmacol Sci* 15: 71–76
24 Maridonneau-Parini I, Errasfa M, Russo-Marie F (1989) Inhibition of O_2^- generation by dexam-
    ethasone is mimicked by lipocortin I in alveolar macrophages. *J Clin Invest* 83: 1936–1940
25 Gold R, Pepinsky RB, Zettl UK, Toyka KV, Hartung HP (1996) Lipocortin-1 (annexin-1) sup-
    presses activation of autoimmune T cell lines in the Lewis rat. *J Neuroimmunol* 69: 157–164

26 Goulding NJ, Pan L, Wardwell K, Guyre VC, Guyre PM (1996) Evidence for specific annexin I-binding proteins on human monocytes. *Biochem J* 316: 593–597
27 Goulding NJ, Pan L, Jefferiss CM, Rigby WFC, Guyre PM (1992) Specific binding of lipocortin 1 (Annexin I) to monocytes and neutrophils is decreased in rheumatoid arthritis. *Arthritis Rheum* 35: 1395–1397
28 Goulding NJ, Guyre PM (1992) Regulation of inflammation by lipocortin I. *Immunol Today* 13: 295–297
29 Karalis K, Crofford LJ, Wilder RL, Chrousos GP (1995) Glucocorticoid and/or glucocorticoid antagonist effects in inflammatory disease-susceptible Lewis rats and inflammatory disease resistant Fischer rats. *Endocrinology* 136: 3107–3112
30 Morand EM, Jefferiss CM, Goulding NJ (1991) Defective corticosteroid induction of lipocortin-1 in rheumatoid leukocytes. *Arthritis Rheum* 34 (Suppl.), S155
31 Podgorski MR, Goulding NJ, Hall ND, Flower RJ, Maddison PJ (1992) Autoantibodies to lipocortin 1 are associated with impaired corticosteroid responsiveness in rheumatoid arthritis. *J Rheumatol* 19: 1668–1671
32 Ikai K, Shimizu K, Kanauchi H, Ando Y, Furukawa F, Imamura S (1992) The presence of autoantibody to lipocortin-I in autoimmune-prone MRL mice. *Autoimmunity* 12: 239
33 Granger DN, Kubes P (1994) The microcirculation and inflammation: modulation of leukocyte-endothelial cell adhesion. *J Leukocyte Biol* 55: 662–675
34 Perretti M, Flower RJ (1996) Measurement of lipocortin 1 levels in murine peripheral blood leukocytes by flow cytometry: modulation by glucocorticoids and inflammation. *Brit J Pharmacol* 118: 605–610
35 Perretti M, Croxtall JD, Wheller SK, Goulding NJ, Hannon R, Flower RJ (1996) Mobilizing lipocortin 1 in adherent human leukocytes downregulates their transmigration. *Nat Med* 2: 1259–1262
36 Goulding NJ (1999) Monitoring steroid responsiveness in RA. *Rheumatology* 38: 907–908
37 Babadjanova G, Allolio B, Vollmer M, Reincke M, Schulte HM (1996) Comparison of the pharmacodynamic effects of deflazacort and prednisolone in healthy subjects. *Eur J Clin Pharmacol* 51: 53–57

Glucocorticoid biology – a historical perspective

Allan Munck

Department of Physiology, Dartmouth Medical School, Lebanon, NH 03756, USA

Introduction

Glucocorticoid biology is a broad and deep subject. Enigmatic as many of their myriad actions may seem, glucocorticoids are undeniably important hormones, since without them most organisms die. They act on almost every cell in the body and are widely used as experimental and therapeutic agents, but even today their physiological functions are hard to define.

The history of glucocorticoids encompasses, among other topics, the discoveries that began a century and a half ago and still continue on the pathology, physiology – including the elusive concept of protection against stress –, chemistry, metabolism, and clinical applications of glucocorticoids; the still sparsely explored roles of glucocorticoids in species beyond a few intensively studied mammals; and the rapidly evolving field, just a few decades old, of mechanisms by which glucocorticoids exert their cellular and molecular actions. The history of each of these topics alone would justify a review or monograph. Here, limited by space and by my knowledge and biases, I will attempt only a brief account, outlining the general history of glucocorticoids up to around 1950, and then bringing a few selected topics up to date. As I proceed, I will refer to books and reviews with more detailed historical information.

Pathological beginnings: Addison's disease and the adrenal glands

Corticosteroids, like many other hormones, first revealed their presence to an astute observer through their absence. Thomas Addison, a physician at Guy's Hospital in London, in 1849, briefly described the symptoms of an almost invariably fatal form of "anemia" that he had observed in a series of patients [1], and added: "In three cases only was there an inspection of the body after death, and in all of them was found a diseased condition of the supra-renal capsules. In two of the cases no disease whatever could be detected in any other part of the body." He tentatively ascribed the cause of the malady to the diseased condition of "these hitherto mysterious bodies – the supra-renal capsules – ...", i.e., the adrenal glands. In a more extensive report on 11 cases [2], he described what came to be known as Addison's Disease: "The leading and characteristic features of the morbid state to which I would direct attention, are, anaemia, general languor and debility, remarkable feebleness of the heart's action, irritability of the stomach, and a peculiar change of colour of the skin, occurring in connection with a diseased condition of the "supra-renal capsules"."

Acceptance of Addison's view of the vital function of the adrenals came slowly, though Brown-Séquard [3] and others soon found that in a number of mammalian species removal of these glands often led rapidly to death. Unsatisfactory experimental techniques and criteria for adrenalectomy, however, gave sufficiently variable results that skepticism about the central role of the adrenals was not dispelled until well into the 20th century [4]. About then it was also established that the life-sustaining functions of the adrenal resided not in the medulla, which was known to produce adrenaline and had already acquired renown through the work of Cannon, but in the cortex [4].

Hormones of the adrenal cortex: glucocorticoids and mineralocorticoids. Cushing's disease and syndrome

Addison's description already foreshadowed some of the stigmata that would eventually be traced to insufficiency of glucocorticoids and mineralocorticoids. Functions of the adrenal cortex first were inferred from the symptoms afflicting Addisonian patients and adrenalectomized animals; then, beginning some 70 years later, from the results of administering adrenal extracts that prolonged life [5, 6]. The functions fell into two main groups: those involving carbohydrate metabolism, in particular maintenance of blood glucose and liver glycogen; and those related to electrolyte and water balance, notably decreased blood concentrations of sodium, chloride and bicarbonate, and increased concentrations of potassium [7]. For a long time one hormone was assumed to be responsible for all these actions [4, 8], but by 1940 results with crystallized extracts from the adrenal cortex revealed at least two distinct types of hormones, later baptized glucocorticoids and mineralocorticoids [9]. Glucocorticoids accounted for effects on carbohydrate metabolism, mineralocorticoids for most effects on electrolyte and water metabolism.

Cushing's disease, the disease of chronic excess of glucocorticoids due to a basophil adenoma in the anterior pituitary, was described some 80 years after Addison's disease [10]. Though rare, it was the model for the set of symptoms known as Cushing's syndrome (weight gain, insulin resistant diabetes, "moon face", "buffalo hump", hypertension, susceptibility to infection, muscular weakness, osteoporosis of the spine, easy bruisability, thin skin), which had been associated with hypersecretion of glucocorticoids [11]. Since 1950, with greatly increased use of glucocorticoids to treat inflammatory and other conditions, Cushing's syndrome has become a common ailment.

Which adrenocortical hormones are essential for life, glucocorticoids or mineralocorticoids?

Even before identification of glucocorticoids and mineralocorticoids, an argument had simmered over which hormonal activity was important for survival. The fact that administration of salt by itself prolonged life [12, 13] supported the role of mineralocorticoid activity, as did reversal of abnormalities of electrolyte balance by adrenal extracts that increased survival. But those extracts also reversed abnormalities of carbohydrate metabolism [14]. Each result was interpreted in favour one or the other activity [15]. Pure steroids settled the matter: both hormonal activities were essential for normal life [15–17].

Important as independent glucocorticoid and mineralocorticoid functions are for mammals, that separation is not universal. It is found in birds and possibly reptiles, but not in fish, where cortisol regulates water and electrolyte as well as carbohydrate metabolism [18, 19].

Physiologists had no trouble understanding why without mineralocorticoids, loss of control of electrolyte and water balance could lead to death. How glucocorticoids sustained life, however, remained unresolved for decades, although it was generally supposed that their effects on carbohydrate metabolism were central to this function [13].

Glucocorticoids and carbohydrate metabolism

Research on the role of glucocorticoids in carbohydrate metabolism intensified during the 1930s. Long and Lukens [20] performed a landmark experiment showing that adrenalectomy is as effective as hypophysectomy in countering diabetes due to pancreatectomy. Their results extended those of Houssay and colleagues who had combined hypophysectomy and pancreatectomy [21], and drew attention to the importance of the adrenal cortex in carbohydrate metabolism. Long, Katzin and Fry [17] in 1940 published a monumental article demonstrating that glucocorticoids stimulate gluconeogenesis from amino acids derived from protein catabolism, decrease glucose oxidation, and can elicit steroid diabetes. Ingle found that glucocorticoids inhibit glucose utilization [22] and cause insulin resistance [23]. These studies laid the foundations for biochemical research in this area [24].

A long-debated question was whether glucocorticoids regulated carbohydrate metabolism by acting directly on peripheral tissues to decrease glucose uptake and release substrates for hepatic gluconeogenesis, or on liver to stimulate gluconeogenesis. Both turned out to be right [24]. Glucocorticoids directly stimulate both hepatic gluconeogenesis and glycogen synthesis. Gluconeogenesis is increased through enhanced activities of the rate-limiting enzymes phosphoenolpyruvate carboxykinase (PEPCK) and glucose-6-phosphatase [25–28]. PEPCK activity is controlled principally through enzyme synthesis [26, 28]; transcription of the PEPCK gene is regulated not only by glucocorticoids but by insulin, glucagon and catecholamines [28]. Increased liver glycogen synthesis was shown to be a direct glucocorticoid effect with fetal liver explants [29]. It is due to increased synthesis and activation of hepatic glycogen synthase [30–32].

Ingle's observations that glucocorticoids inhibit peripheral glucose utilization in whole animals [22], though questioned for some years [24], were eventually confirmed [33–36]. Furthermore, glucocorticoids at physiological concentrations were found to directly inhibit glucose uptake by isolated skin, fibroblasts, adipose cells, lymphocytes, polymorphonuclear leukocytes, and brain cells [24, 37]. Inhibition in adipose cells and fibroblasts due to decreased glucose transport caused by translocation of glucose transporters from the plasma membrane to intracellular sites, the reverse of the action of insulin [38, 39]. Though independent of insulin, the inhibition probably is responsible for significant insulin antagonism [24, 40].

Glucocorticoids also control carbohydrate metabolism in several non-mammalian species, including birds, amphibians, and fish, and may do so in all vertebrates [19]. Detailed mechanisms have not been worked out in these species as they have in mammals.

Pituitary and hypothalamic control of glucocorticoid secretion

Houssay's experiments combining hypophysectomy and pancreatectomy [21] cast light on the role of the pituitary in carbohydrate metabolism and implicated the pituitary in control of the adrenal cortex. Hypophysectomy of several mammalian species as well as of tadpoles and frogs was known by the 1930s to atrophy the adrenal cortex, especially the zonas fasciculata and reticularis [41, 42]. It did not atrophy the zona glomerulasa nor cause disturbances of electrolyte balance such as accompany adrenalectomy. These results therefore showed that the pituitary controlled glucocorticoid secretion from the inner zones, but not mineralocorticoid secretion from the glomerulosa [42–44]. Atrophy of the adrenal cortex could be reversed by pituitary extracts. Such extracts were used to purify the adrenocorticotropic hormone (ACTH) [44–46]. Ingle and Kendall [47] elegantly demonstrated reciprocal control through negative feedback from the adrenals to the pituitary. Stress, known to stimulate the adrenal cortex since the 1930s, was assumed to be transmitted to the adrenals *via* the central nervous system through the pituitary [48], and a hypothalamic factor that stimulated ACTH secretion was postulated by Harris as early as 1937 [49, 50]. After heroic efforts, the corticotropin releasing hormone (CRH) was finally identified in 1981 [51]. Other factors such as vasopressin, catecholamines, and most recently cytokines, are now also known to be important regulators of the hypothalamic-pituitary-adrenal axis [52–55].

Regulation of lymphoid tissue

Hints of adrenal influences on lymphocytes came early. Addison studied the blood of apparently only one of his patients, on whom he reported as follows [2]: "... on subjecting the blood of a patient, who recently died from a well-marked attack of this singular disease, to microscopic examination, a considerable excess of white corpuscles was found to be present." Forty years later Star [56] described an enlarged thymus, " ... as large as that of a child twelve years old", in a patient with Addison's disease. Boinet [57] noted large thymuses in adrenalectomized rats. The converse phenomenon was discovered by Selye, who showed that atrophy of the thymus following injury, toxic substances, and other sources of stress, was mediated by adrenal secretions [58]. Adrenal extracts and pure glucocorticoids caused similar atrophy of the thymus [16, 59, 60] and other lymphoid tissues [61]. Illustrating how easy it is sometimes to mistake cause for effect, early in the 20th century cases of sudden death from unknown causes were sometimes blamed on "Status thymicolymphaticus." This mythical malady was ascribed to a supposedly enlarged thymus by pathologists whose norms for thymus size came from the stress-atrophied thymuses they saw in victims of prolonged illness [62].

The meaning of these glucocorticoid actions began to be understood in the 1960s, when the relation of immunity to lymphoid tissue, and to the thymus in particular, was established [63, 64]. Even today, however, the physiological significance of glucocorticoid-induced lymphocyte death is obscure [65], although the molecular mechanisms of apoptosis [66], the form of programmed cell death by which lymphocytes die, are rapidly being elucidated [67].

A major advance of recent decades was the recognition by Besedovsky, del Rey, Sorkin and colleagues that the immune system is not only a target of glucocorticoids, but can itself stimulate the hypothalamic-pituitary-adrenal axis and increase secretion of glucocorticoids through cytokines like interleukin-1 (IL-1); those cytokines are then suppressed by glucocorticoids, completing a negative feedback loop [54, 68–70].

Anti-inflammatory and immunosuppressive actions

In 1949, the role of glucocorticoids in immune and inflammatory reactions abruptly came to world prominence with the wholly unexpected discovery of the anti-inflammatory actions. Administration of cortisone or ACTH to patients with rheumatoid arthritis was found to cause dramatic improvement [71], and almost overnight glucocorticoids became miracle drugs.

An immediate consequence of this discovery was that clinical demands for glucocorticoids increased astronomically. Hitherto the pharmaceutical industry and organic chemists had been devoted to analyzing and synthesizing adrenal steroids [72, 73] in order to study their physiology and attempt to satisfy the modest clinical needs for treating adrenal insufficiency. Now they rapidly geared up to produce large amounts of cortisone [73, 74] (at the time considered the prototypical glucocorticoid, though later it was realized that for activity, cortisone had to be converted to cortisol [75]). They also developed synthetic analogs of glucocorticoids with reduced unwanted side-effects like salt retention and feedback suppression. During the 1950s these efforts produced many of the glucocorticoids still in use, such as prednisone, prednisolone, dexamethasone, and triamcinolone [76, 77].

Immunosuppression soon emerged as an unwanted side-effect when patients treated with glucocorticoids for inflammatory conditions became immunosuppressed and susceptible to infection [78, 79]. But soon it became a potential asset when glucocorticoids were found to prolong survival of skin grafts [80, 81]. Eventually glucocorticoid actions on inflammatory and immune reactions were recognized to be so closely related as to be almost inseparable, sharing cellular and molecular mechanisms involving control of cytokines, prostaglandins, and other mediators [82–84].

As described below, although for decades after their discovery the anti-inflammatory and immunosuppressive actions were believed by physiologists to have no physiological significance [44], these actions are now accepted as essential physiological components of glucocorticoid-mediated resistance to stress [65, 85–87].

Resistance to stress: regulatory and permissive actions

Already by 1930 it was evident that adrenalectomized animals and patients with Addison's disease were extremely sensitive to stress induced by a wide range of challenges to homeostasis (toxins, infections, trauma, heat, cold, strenuous exercise, fear, and many others), and that adrenal extracts conferred resistance to such "stressors" [5, 15, 88, 89]. Selye, who contributed many studies on stress and popularized use of the term well beyond endocrinology [48, 58, 90, 91], developed a theoretical framework for the role of the adrenal cortex which introduced such concepts as "the alarm reaction", "the general adaptation syndrome", "diseases of adaptation", and "adaptation energy". Although these terms have fallen into disuse, Selye stimulated thinking and generated vigorous debates on the subject of corticosteroids and stress. Perhaps his most lasting contribution was to emphasize that all stressors elicited a stereotyped set of nonspecific responses, "the alarm reaction", central to which was increased secretion of adrenocortical hormones [48]. Swingle and coworkers found that among these hormones glucocorticoids were the most effective in conferring resistance to stress, and concluded that adrenalectomized animals were weakened by a failure of intermediate metabolism [13].

Implicit in most thinking on how stress-elevated levels of glucocorticoids conferred resistance to stress was the plausible assumption that they enhanced the capacity of the body's defense mechanisms to cope with stress [79, 85].

Along these lines, Selye proposed that stress-induced glucocorticoids protect through their effects on carbohydrate metabolism, increasing energy supplies to the body in the form of glucose [48]. This idea has not survived, since glucose alone cannot replace glucocorticoids [92, 93].

Another suggestion that held sway for some time [4] was that of White and colleagues [94], who claimed that stress-induced levels of adrenocortical hormones released antibodies from lysed lymphocytes, thereby furnishing rapid resistance to infection. This work could not be confirmed, however [44, 95, 96].

A different slant on how glucocorticoids protect came from the work of Ingle [92, 97]. He found that adrenalectomized animals resist certain forms of stress even if given glucocorticoids only at basal replacement levels. He concluded that such "permissive" effects, as he called them, suffice to maintain the organism's responsiveness to moderate stress, whereas the "regulatory" effects of high, stress-induced glucocorticoid levels emphasized by Selye are required for resistance to severe stress [97].

Stress and the anti-inflammatory actions

Discovery of the anti-inflammatory actions caused turmoil among glucocorticoid physiologists, particularly over the question of how stress-induced glucocorticoids protect against stress. As discussed in more detail elsewhere [85], physiologists were unable to provide a physiological explanation for anti-inflammatory actions, which were inconsistent with their assumption that glucocorticoids stimulated defense mechanisms [79]. As a result, interest in how glucocorticoids protected against stress gradually dissipated. Selye's theory of diseases of adaptation, according to which collagen diseases like rheumatoid arthritis were caused by excessive amounts of adrenal steroids, also suffered a decline, since anti-inflammatory actions demonstrated the opposite [44, 74].

Physiologists tried to deal with those contradictions by dismissing anti-inflammatory and related actions of glucocorticoids as pharmacological, not physiological [15, 44]. That view, despite a rare voice to the contrary [79], persisted up to the 1980s, and the spectacular rise in therapeutic applications of glucocorticoids proceeded largely without participation of physiologists. Their state of mind is illustrated by several influential reviews from that period on the role of the adrenal cortex in homeostasis and stress [92, 98, 99]: none of them refer to any work on anti-inflammatory actions.

As more and more observations were made on glucocorticoid actions in whole animals and isolated tissues and cells, however, the notion that anti-inflammatory and other suppressive actions had nothing to do with physiology became untenable [85]. For example, numerous glucocorticoid effects underlying immunosuppressive actions, such as inhibition of cytokine secretion, were elicited in isolated cells with physiological glucocorticoid concentrations, indicating that they probably occurred under normal physiological conditions in intact organisms (as many of them were eventually shown to do [83]). Furthermore, most effects of glucocorticoids in isolated systems were turning out to be suppressive [85].

Roles of glucocorticoids in stress

The question, then, was how to reconcile these predominantly suppressive influences of glucocorticoids with their protective roles in stress. My colleagues and I proposed in 1984 that stress-induced glucocorticoids, rather than stimulate defense mechanisms, suppressed them in order to prevent them from overshooting and damaging the organism [85]. We originally gathered substantial evidence for this hypothesis, and more has appeared since [65, 83]. So far, no fatal flaws have been identified. The strength of the hypothesis was that it offered reasonable physiological functions for anti-inflammatory and other suppressive actions of stress-induced glucocorticoids. Also, by removing the "pharmacological" stigma physiologists had placed on those actions, it opened the door to reunifying glucocorticoid endocrinology.

Having found no antecedents in the endocrine literature for our hypothesis, we believed it was new. We were mistaken, however. In germinal form, it had been proposed many years earlier by Marius Tausk [79]. Tausk, a physician and co-managing director of the Dutch pharmaceutical firm Organon, in 1951, published a review on the recently discovered anti-inflammatory actions of glucocorticoids. Trying to make physiological sense of those actions in the context of Selye's ideas, he tentatively suggested essentially the hypothesis just described, epitomizing the role of glucocorticoids in stress as like that of preventing water damage caused by firefighters extinguishing a fire. The review appeared in an Organon journal distributed mainly for the benefit of practicing physicians. Tausk's idea apparently never entered the regular endocrine literature, and did not come to the notice of most glucocorticoid physiologists. There is no mention of it in any of the influential reviews referred to earlier. Had it received wider attention, glucocorticoid physiology might have followed a more constructive course than the one embarked on in 1950.

Permissive actions of glucocorticoids at basal levels [92, 97], which can be thought of as "priming" certain defense mechanisms for action, play important complementary roles to the suppressive actions. As can be illustrated by a simple mathematical model, when permissive and suppressive actions are linked they considerably extend the range of glucocorticoid effectiveness [83, 100].

Ottaviani and Franceschi [101] have reviewed the neuroimmunology of stress from invertebrates to man, emphasizing how widely applicable is Selye's notion of a stereotyped stress-response. Wendelaar Bonga [18] has described the mechanisms of stress in fish *via* the hypothalamic-pituitary-interrenal axis (interrenals being the corticosteroid-producing cells in fish), and the numerous functions of cortisol. The many roles of glucocorticoids in stress, including permissive, suppressive, and other actions, have recently been analyzed in a broad ethological setting [65].

Cellular and molecular mechanisms of action of glucocorticoids

Research on cellular and molecular mechanisms of action of glucocorticoids and other steroid hormones has a short but intense history. Up through the 1950s, studies with steroid hormones established a number of potential target tissues, such as the liver and thymus for glucocorticoids and the uterus for estrogens, but no direct effects have been demonstrated on isolated tissues and cells by addition of steroid hormones at physiological concentrations. In retrospect, at least two obstacles hindered progress: the slowness of the actions of these hormones, which required long incubations not well tolerated by freshly isolated cells and tissues (in those days few cell lines were available); and the ease with which nonspecific effects of steroid hormones could be obtained rapidly on isolated tissues, cells, and even pure enzymes, simply by using high enough steroid concentrations. Effects of steroid hormones at 10^{-4} M, such as were regularly reported, were probably attributable to their interfacial activities [102]. Nonspecific steroid effects of this kind, devoid of physiological significance, beguiled and misled researchers for years.

Finally, in the 1960s, the first direct effects of steroid hormones at physiological concentrations on isolated systems were demonstrated. Overell, Condon and Petrow showed that glucocorticoids inhibit glucose uptake by isolated skin [103], and my colleagues and I found they inhibit glucose uptake by adipose tissue [104, 105] and thymus cells [35]. These observations agreed well with effects seen in whole animals [22, 24, 33, 105, 106]. Once the floodgates opened many other cells were found to respond directly to glucocorticoids, and eventually, to have glucocorticoid receptors [107].

A curious note from the 1950s and 60s is that, until the model of receptor-mediated genomic actions took over, the most widely discussed mechanisms of steroid hormone action had no receptors, but invoked special properties of the steroid molecules themselves to account for hormone specificity. For example, Talalay and Williams-Ashman showed that pairs of steroids like estradiol and estrone, which could exchange a hydrogen at carbon-17, catalyzed transhydrogenation between NADP and NAD by serving as coenzymes in the reversible transfer of hydrogen, using a hydroxysteroid dehydrogenase possessing dual pyridine nucleotide specificity [108–110]. They suggested that such a mechanism might account for actions of other steroid hormones. This ingenious idea foundered on the demonstration by Jensen and Jacobsen that no exchange of the hydrogen atom at C-17 occurs in receptor-bound estradiol [111]. Yielding and Tomkins [112] observed that various steroid hormones inhibit the activity and alter the structure of pure glutamic dehydrogenase in solution, through what later would be known as allosteric interactions. Their proposal that these results were examples of physiological hormone action were unconvincing, however, because of the high hormone concentrations required and the poor correlation with hormonal activity. Willmer [113], impressed by the similarities between the steroid hormones and cholesterol and by evidence for the interfacial activity of steroid hormones [114], suggested that the hormones act by intercalating into cell membranes and modulating membrane functions. This mechanism never received significant experimental support, but is reincarnated in today's much more firmly based ideas on nongenomic steroid hormone actions *via* membrane receptors [115].

Our metabolic studies with rat thymus cells led us to glucocorticoid receptors [116, 117]. By then estrogen receptors had been discovered by Jensen and Jacobson [111, 118], who observed retention of radioactive estradiol in presumed estrogen target tissues like the uterus, and mineralocorticoid receptors had been discovered by Edelman, Bogorosh and Porter [119], who used autoradiography to demonstrate saturable binding of radioactive aldosterone in toad bladder cells. We incubated thymus cells with radioactive steroids (tritiated cortisol was initially our probe) under conditions similar to those we used to elicit metabolic effects; then we measured their dissociation rates. That procedure allowed us to separate the large non-specifically bound steroid fraction that dissociated rapidly, from the smaller receptor-bound steroid fraction that dissociated relatively slowly. Our principal criteria for glucocorticoid receptors were that their affinities for natural and synthetic glucocorticoids should be roughly proportional to the biological activities of the steroids in the thymus cells, and that binding to the receptors should precede the earliest detectable metabolic effects. From a historical point of view, an interesting if peripheral result was that cortisone, long considered the prototypical glucocorticoid, was neither metabolically active nor bound to the receptors in thymus cells [117], confirming a prediction by Bush [75]. Using a somewhat similar method Schaumburg and Bojesen [120] independently identified glucocorticoid receptors in rat thymus cells. The dissociation method, though invaluable for our initial explorations, was soon replaced by simpler methods that measured saturable binding of synthetic glucocorticoids like dexamethasone and triamcinolone acetonide.

Glucocorticoid receptors were found in cultured fibroblasts by Pratt, Hackney, Aronow and colleagues [121–123], and in hepatoma and lymphoma cells by Baxter, Tomkins, Rousseau, and coworkers [124–127]. These studies initiated use of cell lines for investigating receptors. When liver and other normal tissues were studied, glucocorticoid receptors turned up everywhere [107, 128–130]. Brain binding sites for corticosterone identified by McEwen and coworkers [131] were later shown to belong to mineralocorticoid receptors [132].

One of the most startling turnabouts in glucocorticoid and mineralocorticoid history was the discovery that cortisol and corticosterone (the natural glucocorticoids), contrary to earlier evidence, had much higher affinity for mineralocorticoid than for glucocorticoid receptors [133]. The puzzle of how aldosterone bound to mineralocorticoid receptors in the face of much higher concentrations of glucocorticoids (which bound with an affinity comparable to that of aldosterone) was resolved by the discovery that mineralocorticoid target tissues have high levels of the enzyme 11β-hydroxysteroid dehydrogenase Type II which "protects" mineralocorticoid receptors. It inactivates cortisol and corticosterone, converting them to cortisone and 11-dehydrocorticosterone [134, 135]. Probably some glucocorticoid actions in the brain and elsewhere are mediated by mineralocorticoid receptors [65, 132]. Certain glucocorticoid receptors may be protected from glucocorticoids by the same enzyme [136].

In the early days of receptor research there was little anticipation of the profound similarities that would emerge between all steroid hormone receptors (and ultimately between all the so-called nuclear receptors of the steroid-thyroid-retinoid superfamily). But as the various receptors were purified and characterized it became clear that they shared numerous characteristics, such as that they were proteins of comparable sizes, and dissociated into smaller components when "activated" or "transformed" by hormone binding at 37 °C [137]. Detailed studies by Pratt, Toft, Gehring and others have led to a model in which the unliganded receptor forms a large heterocomplex with heat shock and other proteins [137, 138]. On hormone binding the heterocomplex dissociates, producing a hormone-receptor complex with high affinity for nuclear sites associated with target genes. The receptor is then recycled and reutilized *via* ATP-dependent steps [137].

One of the most significant common properties of steroid hormone receptors was discerned at the cellular level. All the receptors, including the glucocorticoid receptor [139–141], bound in the nuclei of their target cells after treatment with hormone. Cell fractionation studies that placed all unliganded receptors in the cytoplasm turned out to be wrong. Immunocytochemical and other techniques later showed that except for glucocorticoid and mineralocorticoid receptors, all the receptors are predominantly nuclear even in unliganded form, becoming bound to chromatin only after hormone binding. The different localizations of the unliganded receptors may not have deep significance since receptors probably traffic constantly between cytoplasm and nucleus [137].

Hormone-induced binding of receptors in the nucleus was consistent with the model of genomic regulation by steroid hormones developed through the 1960s. In today's model of receptor-mediated genomic control, each steroid hormone binds to its specific intracellular receptors to form hormone-receptor complexes that associate with and regulate transcription of target genes. That model began to take shape in the 1950s. By the early 1970s it had swept the field. Its origins can be traced back to insect physiology, particularly to the work of Wigglesworth [142], Schneiderman and Gilbert [143], and Karlson [144]. The observation that the prothoracic gland hormone ecdysone (which structurally resembles the steroid hormones) caused chromosome puffing associated with RNA synthesis, led them to consider that this hormone exerted its developmental effects through activation of transcription of certain genes. Karlson extended this idea to glucocorticoids and other hormones

[144]. At that time Knox had already provided strong evidence that in the liver, glucocorticoids induce synthesis of certain enzymes [145, 146].

After those first stirrings, innumerable experiments were done to show that glucocorticoid and other steroid hormone actions could be blocked with inhibitors of protein synthesis like puromycin, and inhibitors of RNA synthesis like actinomycin D [107]. Eventually, more direct evidence began to come in for induction of synthesis of mRNA and proteins. Progress since then has gone hand-in-hand with advances in molecular biology.

A major breakthrough came in the 1980s with the cloning of glucocorticoid and other steroid hormone receptors, which revealed their common domain structures [147–149]. Another came with the identification of glucocorticoid response elements (GREs) associated with target genes. Together, these findings began to show how glucocorticoid receptors regulate gene transcription [148, 150, 151]. During the 1990s the convergence of investigations on structure and function has continued apace, to the point where it seems not unrealistic to think that within some years, the molecular interactions initiating a steroid hormone effect may be visualized at the atomic level [152, 153]. Recent studies with transgenic mice in which glucocorticoid receptors have been knocked out or modified [154, 155], raise hopes that it will ultimately be possible to link the deep insights on primary molecular mechanisms to the physiology of glucocorticoids that has preoccupied physicians and scientists for 150 years.

References

1 Addison T (1849). Anæmia – disease of the supra-renal capsules. *London Medical Gazette* 43: 517–518
2 Addison T (1855). *On the constitutional and local effects of disease of the suprarenal capsules.* Highley, London
3 Brown-Séquard CE (1856). Recherches expérimentales sur la physiologie et la pathologie des capsules surrénales. *Compt Rend Soc Biol* 43: 422–425
4 Gaunt R, Eversole WJ (1949) Notes on the history of the adrenocortical problem. *Ann N Y Acad Sci* 50: 511–521
5 Hartman FA, Brownell KA, Hartman WE (1930) A further study of the hormone of the adrenal cortex. *Amer J Physiol* 95: 670–680
6 Swingle WW, Pfiffner JJ (1931) Studies on the adrenal cortex. I. The effect of a lipid fraction upon the life-span of adrenalectomized cats. *Amer J Physiol* 96: 153–163
7 Loeb RF, Atchley DW, Benedict EM, Leland J (1933) Electrolyte balance studies in adrenalectomized dogs with particular reference to excretion of sodium. *J Exp Med* 57: 775
8 Hartman FA, Brownell KA (1930) The hormone of the adrenal cortex. *Science* 72: 76
9 Selye H (1947) *Textbook of endocrinology.* Acta Endocrinologica, Montreal
10 Cushing H (1932) The basophil adenomas of the pituitary body and their clinical manifestations (pituitary basophilism). *Bull Johns Hopkins Hosp* 50: 137–195
11 Albright F (1943) Cushing's Syndrome. Its relationship to the adrenogenital syndrome, and its connection with the problem of the reaction of the body to injurious agents ("Alarm Reaction" of Selye). *Harvey Lectures* 38: 123–186
12 Loeb RF (1933) Effect of sodium chloride treatment of a patient with Addison's disease. *Proc Soc Exp Biol Med* 30: 808
13 Swingle WW, Remington JW (1944) The role of the adrenal cortex in physiological processes. *Physiol Rev* 24: 89

14 Britton SW, Silvette H (1932) The apparent prepotent function of the adrenal glands. *Amer J Physiol* 100: 701–713
15 Gaunt R (1975) History of the adrenal cortex. *In*: H Blaschko, G Sayers, AD Smith (eds): *Handbook of Physiology.* Physiology Society, Washington, D.C., 1–12
16 Wells BB, Kendall EC (1940) A qualitative difference in the effect of compounds separated from the adrenal cortex on distribution of electrolytes and on atrophy of the adrenal and thymus glands of rats. *Proc Mayo Clin* 15: 133–139
17 Long CNH, Katzin B, Fry EG (1940) The adrenal cortex and carbohydrate metabolism. *Endocrinology* 26: 309–344
18 Wendelaar Bonga SE (1997) The stress response in fish. *Physiol Rev* 77: 591–625
19 Bentley PJ (1998) *Comparative Vertebrate Endocrinology,* 3rd ed. Cambridge University Press, Cambridge, England
20 Long CNH, Lukens FDW (1936) The effects of adrenalectomy and hypophysectomy upon experimental diabetes in the cat. *J Exp Med* 63: 465–490
21 Houssay BA, Biasotti A (1931) The hypophysis, carbohydrate metabolism and diabetes. *Endocrinology* 15: 511–523
22 Ingle DJ (1941) The production of glycosuria in the normal rat by means of 17-hydroxy-11-dehydrocorticosterone. *Endocrinology* 29: 649–652
23 Ingle DJ, Sheppard R, Evans JS, Kuizenga MH (1945) A comparison of adrenal steroid diabetes and pancreatic diabetes in the rat. *Endocrinology* 37: 341–356
24 Munck A (1971) Glucocorticoid inhibition of glucose uptake by peripheral tissues: old and new evidence, molecular mechanisms, and physiological significance. *Perspect Biol Med* 14: 265–289
25 Shrago E, Lardy HA, Nordlie RC, Foster DO (1963) Metabolic and hormonal control of phosphoenolpyruvate carboxykinase and malic enzyme in rat liver. *J Biol Chem* 238: 3188–3192
26 Exton JH (1979) Regulation of gluconeogenesis by glucocorticoids. *In*: JD Baxter, GG Rousseau (eds): *Glucocorticoid hormone action.* Springer, Berlin, 535–546
27 Exton JH (1987) Mechanisms of hormonal regulation of hepatic glucose metabolism. *Diab Metab Rev* 3: 163–183
28 Pilkis SJ, Granner DK (1992) Molecular physiology of the regulation of hepatic gluconeogenesis and glycolysis. *Annu Rev Physiol* 54: 885–909
29 Monder C, Coufalik A (1972) Influence of cortisol on glycogen synthesis and gluconeogenesis in fetal rat liver in organ culture. *J Biol Chem* 247: 3608–3617
30 von Holt C, Fister J (1964) The effect of cortisol on synthesis and degradation of liver glycogen. *Biochim Biophys Acta* 90: 232–238
31 Hornbrook KR, Burch HB, Lowry OH (1966) The effects of adrenalectomy and hydrocortisone on rat liver metabolites and glycogen synthetase activity. *Mol Pharmacol* 2: 106–116
32 Bollen M, Stalmans W (1992) The structure, role, and regulation of type 1 protein phosphatases. *Crit Rev Biochem Molec Biol* 27: 227–281
33 Munck A, Koritz SB (1962) Studies on the mode of action of glucocorticoids in rats. I. Early effects of cortisol on blood glucose and on glucose entry into muscle, liver and adipose tissue. *Biochim Biophys Acta* 57: 310–317
34 Riddick FA, Reisler DM, Kipnis DM (1962) The sugar transport system in striated muscle. Effect of growth hormone, hydrocortisone and alloxan diabetes. *Diabetes* 11: 171–178
35 Morita Y, Munck A (1964) Effect of glucocorticoids *in vivo* and *in vitro* on net glucose uptake and amino acid incorporation by rat-thymus cells. *Biochim Biophys Acta* 93: 150–157
36 Doyle P, Guillaume-Gentile C, Rohner-Jeanrenaud F, Jeanrenaud B (1994) Effects of corticosterone administration on local cerebral glucose utilization of rats. *Brain Res* 645: 225
37 Horner H, Packan D, Sapolsky R (1990) Glucocorticoids inhibit glucose transport in cultured hippocampal neurons and glia. *Neuroendocrinology* 52: 57–63
38 Carter-Su C, Okamoto K (1985) Effect of glucocorticoids on hexose transport in rat adipocytes: evidence for decreased transporters in the plasma membrane. *J Biol Chem* 260: 11091–11098
39 Horner HC, Munck A, Lienhard GE (1987) Dexamethasone causes translocation of glucose transporters from the plasma membrane to an intracellular site in human fibroblasts. *J Biol Chem* 262: 17696–17702
40 McMahon M, Gerich J, Rizza R (1988) Effects of glucocorticoids on carbohydrate metabolism. *Diab Metab Rev* 4: 17–30
41 Swann HG (1940) The pituitary-adrenocortical relationship. *Physiol Rev* 20: 493–521
42 Chester Jones I (1957) *The Adrenal Cortex.* Cambridge University Press, Cambridge, England

43 Smith PE (1930) Hypophysectomy and a replacement therapy in the rat. *Amer J Anat* 45: 205–273
44 Sayers G (1950) The adrenal cortex and homeostasis. *Physiol Rev* 30: 241–320
45 Li CH, Evans HM, Simpson ME (1943) Adrenocorticotropic hormone. *J Biol Chem* 149: 413–424
46 Sayers G, White A, Long CNH (1943) Preparation and properties of adrenotropic hormone. *J Biol Chem* 149: 425–436
47 Ingle DJ, Kendall EC (1937) Atrophy of the adrenal cortex of the rat produced by the administration of large amounts of cortin. *Science* 86: 245
48 Selye H (1946) The general adaptation syndrome and the diseases of adaptation. *J Clin Endocrinol Metab* 6: 117–230
49 Harris GW (1937) The induction of ovulation in the rabbit, by electrical stimulation of the hypothalamo-hypophysial mechanism. *Proc R Soc Lond B* 122: 374–394
50 Harris GW (1955) *Neural Control of the Pituitary Gland.* Edward Arnold, London
51 Vale W, Spiess J, Rivier C, Rivier J (1981) Characterization of a 41-residue ovine hypothalamic peptide that stimulates secretion of corticotropin and β-endorphin. *Science* 213: 1394
52 Tilders FJH, Berkenbosch F, Vermes I, Linton EA, Smelik PG (1985) Role of epinephrine and vasopressin in the control of the pituitary-adrenal response to stress. *Federation Proc* 44: 155–160
53 Dallman MF, Akana SF, Cascio CS, Darlington DN, Jacobson L, Levin N (1987) Regulation of ACTH secretion: variations on a theme of B. *Recent Prog Horm Res* 43: 113–173
54 Besedovsky HO, del Rey A, Klusman I, Furukawa H, Arditi GM, Kabiersch A (1991) Cytokines as modulators of the hypothalamus-pituitary-adrenal axis. *J Steroid Biochem Molec Biol* 40: 613–618
55 Turnbull AV, Rivier C (1996) Corticotropin-releasing factor, vasopressin, and prostaglandins mediate, and nitric oxide restrains, the hypothalamic-pituitary-adrenal response to acute local inflammation in the rat. *Endocrinology* 137: 455–463
56 Star P (1895). An unusual case of Addison's disease; sudden death; remarks. *Lancet* 284
57 Boinet E (1899). Recherches expérimentales sur les fonctions des capsules surrénales. *Compt Rend Soc Biol* 51: 671–672
58 Selye H (1936) Thymus and adrenals in the response of the organism to injuries and intoxications. *Brit J ExpPathol* 17: 234–248
59 Ingle DJ (1938) Atrophy of the thymus in normal and hypophysectomized rats following administration of cortin. *Proc Soc Exp Biol Med* 38: 443–444
60 Ingle DJ (1940) Effect of two steroid compounds on weight of thymus of adrenalectomized rats. *Proc Soc Exp Biol Med* 44: 174–175
61 Dougherty TF (1952) Effect of hormones on lymphatic tissues. *Physiol Rev* 32: 379–401
62 Greenwood M, Woods HM (1927) "Status thymico-lymphaticus" considered in the light of recent work on the thymus. *J Hygiene* 26: 305–326
63 Miller JFAP (1967) Current concepts of the immunological function of the thymus. *Physiol Rev* 47: 437–520
64 Gowans JL (1968) Lymphocytes. *Harvey Lectures* 64
65 Sapolsky RM, Romero LM, Munck A (2000). How do glucocorticoids influence stress-responses? Integrating permissive, suppressive, stimulatory, and preparative actions. *Endocrin Rev* 21: 55–89
66 Kerr JFR, Wyllie AH, Currie AR (1972) Apoptosis: a basic biological phenomenon with wide-ranging implications in tissue kinetics. *Brit J Cancer* 26: 239–257
67 Vaux DL, Korsmeyer SJ (1999) Cell death in development. *Cell* 96: 245–254
68 Besedovsky H, Sorkin E, Keller M, Müller J (1975) Changes in blood hormone levels during the immune response. *Proc Soc Exp Biol Med* 150: 466–470
69 Besedovsky H, Sorkin E (1977) Network of immune-neuroendocrine interactions. *Clin Exp Immunol* 27: 1–12
70 Besedovsky HO, del Rey A (1996) Immuno-neuro-endocrine interactions: facts and hypotheses. *Endocrin Rev* 17: 64–102
71 Hench PS, Kendall EC, Slocumb CH, Polley HF (1949) The effect of a hormone of the adrenal cortex (17-hydroxy-11-dehydrocorticosterone: compound E) and of pituitary adrenocorticotropic hormone on rheumatoid arthritis. *Proc Mayo Clin* 24: 181–197
72 Kendall EC (1949) The chemistry and partial synthesis of adrenal steroids. *Ann N Y Acad Sci* 50
73 Wettstein A (1954) Adv. the field of adrenal cortical hormones. *Experientia* 10: 397–416
74 Kendall EC (1971) *Cortisone.* Charles Scribner's Sons, New York
75 Bush IE (1962) Chemical and biological factors in the activity of adrenocortical steroids.

Pharmacol Rev 14: 317–445

76 Fried J, Borman A (1958) Synthetic derivatives of cortical hormones. Vitam Hormone 16: 303–374

77 Sarett LH (1959) Some aspects of the evolution of anti-inflammatory steroids. Ann N Y Acad Sci 82: 802–808

78 Editorial (1950) Cortisone and A.C.T.H. in tuberculosis. Lancet 632

79 Tausk M (1951) Hat die Nebenniere tatsächlich eine Verteidigungsfunktion? Das Hormon (Organon,Holland) 3: 1–24

80 Billingham RE, Krohn PL, Medawar PB (1951) Effect of cortisone on survival of skin homografts in rabbits. Brit Med J 1: 1157–1163

81 Medawar PB, Sparrow EM (1956) The effects of adrenocortical hormones, adrenocorticotrophic hormone and pregnancy on skin transplantation immunity in mice. J Endocrinol 14: 240–256

82 Goldstein RA, Bowen DL, Fauci AS (1992) Adrenal Corticosteroids. In: JI Gallin, IM Goldstein, R Snyderman (eds): Inflammation. Basic Principles and Clinical Correlates. Raven Press, New York, 1061–1081

83 Munck A, Náray-Fejes-Tóth A (1994) Glucocorticoids and stress: permissive and suppressive actions. Ann N Y Acad Sci 746: 115–130

84 Goulding NJ (1998) Corticosteroids – a case of mistaken identity. Brit J Rheumatol 37: 477–483

85 Munck A, Guyre PM, Holbrook NJ (1984) Physiological functions of glucocorticoids in stress and their relation to pharmacological actions. Endocrin Rev 5: 25–44

86 Sternberg EM, Hill JM, Chrousos GP, Kamilaris T, Listwak SJ, Gold PW, Wilder RL (1989) Inflammatory mediator-induced hypothalamic-pituitary-adrenal axis activation is defective in streptococcal cell wall arthritis-susceptible Lewis rats. Proc Natl Acad Sci USA 86: 2374–2378

87 Derijk R, Berkenbosch F (1991) The immune-hypothalamo-pituitary-adrenal axis and autoimmunity. Int J Neurosci 59: 91–100

88 Scott WJM (1923) The influence to the adrenal glands on resistance. I. The susceptibility of adrenalectomized rats to morphine. J Exp Med xxxviii: 543–560

89 Ingle DJ (1942) Problems relating to the adrenal cortex. Endocrinology 31: 419–438

90 Selye H (1937) The significance of the adrenals for adaptation. Science 85: 247–248

91 Selye H (1956) The Stress of Life. McGraw-Hill, New York

92 Ingle DJ (1952) The role of the adrenal cortex in homeostasis. J Endocrinol 8, xxiii–xxxvii

93 Darlington DN, Chew G, Ha T, Keil LC, Dallman MF (1990) Corticosterone, but not glucose, treatment enables fasted adrenalectomized rats to survive moderate hemorrhage. Endocrinology 127: 766–772

94 White A, Dougherty TF (1945) The pituitary adrenotrophic hormone control of the rate of release of serum globulins from lymphoid tissue. Endocrinology 36: 207–217

95 Eisen HN, Mayer MM, Moore DH, Tarr R-R, Stoerk HC (1947) Failure of adrenal cortical activity to influence circulating antibodies and gamma globulin. Proc Soc Exp Biol Med 65: 301–306

96 Waksman BH (1985) Neuroimmunomodulation of homeostasis and host defense. J Immunol 135: 862s

97 Ingle DJ (1954) Permissibility of hormone action. A review. Acta Endocrinol 17: 172–186

98 Hoffman FG (1971) Role of the adrenal cortex in homeostasis and growth. In: NP Christy (ed.): The human adrenal cortex. Harper and Row, New York, 303–316

99 Selye H (1971) Hormones and resistance. J Pharmacol Sci 60: 1–28

100 Munck A, Náray-Fejes-Tóth A (1992) The ups and downs of glucocorticoid physiology. Permissive and suppressive effects revisited. Mol Cell Endocrinol 90, C1–C4

101 Ottaviani E, Franceschi C (1996) The neuroimmunology of stress from invertebrates to man. Prog Neurobiol 48: 421–440

102 Engel LL (1961) Discussion. In: CA Villee, LL Engel (eds): Mechanism of action of adrenal cortical hormones. Pergamon Press, New York, 85–86 107–109

103 Overell BG, Condon SE, Petrow V (1960) The effect of hormones and their analogues upon the uptake of glucose by mouse skin in vitro. J Pharm Pharmacol 12: 150–153

104 Munck A (1961) The effect in vitro of glucocorticoids on net glucose uptake by rat epididymal adipose tissue. Biochim Biophys Acta 48: 618–620

105 Munck A (1962) Studies on the mode of action of glucocorticoids in rats. II. The effects in vivo and in vitro on net glucose uptake by isolated adipose tissue. Biochim Biophys Acta 57: 318–326

106 Bartlett D, Morita Y, Munck A (1962) Rapid inhibition by cortisol of incorporation of glucose in vivo into the thymus of the rat. Nature 196: 897–898

107 Munck A, Leung K (1977) Glucocorticoid receptors and mechanisms of action. *In*: JR Pasqualini (ed.): *Receptors and mechanism of action of steroid hormones, Part II*. Marcel Dekker, New York, 311–397

108 Talalay P, Hurlock B, Williams-Ashman HG (1959) On a coenzymatic function of estradiol-17beta. *Proc Natl Acad Sci USA* 44

109 Hurlock B, Talalay P (1958) 3α -hydroxysteroids as coenzymes of hydrogen transfer between di- and triphosphopyridine nucleotides. *J Biol Chem* 233: 886–893

110 Laidler KJ, Krupka RM (1961) Enzyme mechanisms in relation to the mode of action of steroid hormones. *In*: CA Villee, LL Engel (eds): *Mechanism of action of steroid hormones*. Pergamon Press, New York, 235–246

111 Jensen EV, Jacobson HI (1962) Basic guides to the mechanism of estrogen action. *Recent Prog Horm Res* 18: 387–414

112 Yielding KL, Tomkins GM (1960) Structural alterations in crystalline glutamic dehydrogenase induced by steroid hormones. *Proc Soc Natl Acad Sci USA* 46

113 Willmer EN (1961) Steroids and cell surfaces. *Biol Rev* 36: 368–398

114 Munck A (1957) The interfacial activity of steroid hormones and synthetic estrogens. *Biochim Biophys Acta* 24: 507–514

115 Wehling H (1997) Specific, nongenomic actions of steroid hormones. *Annu Rev Physiol* 59: 365–393

116 Munck A, Brinck-Johnsen T (1967) Specific metabolic and physicochemical interactions of glucocorticoids *in vivo* and *in vitro* with rat adipose tissue and thymus cells. *Excerpta Medica Int Cong Ser* 132: 472–481

117 Munck A, Brinck-Johnsen T (1968) Specific and nonspecific physicochemical interactions of glucocorticoids and related steroids with rat thymus cells *in vitro*. *J Biol Chem* 243: 5556–5565

118 Jensen EV (1991) Steroid hormone receptors. *In*: G Seifert (ed.): *Current topics in pathology, vol. 83, cell receptors*. Springer, Berlin, 365–431

119 Edelman IS, Bogorosh R, Porter GA (1963) On the mechanism of action of aldosterone on sodium transport: the role of protein synthesis. *Proc Natl Acad Sci USA* 50: 1169–1177

120 Schaumburg BP, Bojesen E (1968) Specificity and thermodynamic properties of the corticosteroid binding to a receptor of rat thymocytes *in vitro*. *Biochim Biophys Acta* 170: 172–188

121 Hackney JF, Gross SR, Aronow L, Pratt WB (1970) Specific glucocorticoid-binding macromolecules from mouse fibroblasts growing *in vitro*. A possible steroid receptor for growth inhibition. *Mol Pharmacol* 6: 500–512

122 Hackney JF, Pratt WB (1971) Characterization and partial purification of the specific glucocorticoid-binding component from mouse fibroblasts. *Biochemistry* 10: 3002–3008

123 Ishii DN, Pratt WB, Aronow L (1972) Steady-state level of the specific glucocorticoid binding component in mouse fibroblasts. *Biochemistry* 11: 3896–3904

124 Baxter JD, Tomkins GM (1970) The relationship between glucocorticoid binding and tyrosine aminotrasferase induction in hepatoma tissue culture cells. *Proc Natl Acad Sci USA* 65: 709–715

125 Baxter JD, Tomkins GM (1971) Specific cytoplasmic glucocorticoid hormone receptors in hepatoma tissue culture cells. *Proc Natl Acad Sci USA* 68: 932–937

126 Baxter JD, Harris AW, Tomkins GM, Cohn M (1971) Glucocorticoid receptors in lymphoma cells in culture: relationship to glucocorticoid killing activity. *Science* 171: 189–191

127 Rousseau GG, Baxter JD, Tomkins GM (1972) Glucocorticoid receptors: relations between steroid binding and biological effects. *J Mol Biol* 67: 99–115

128 Beato M, Kalimi M, Feigelson P (1972) Correlation between glucocorticoid binding to specific liver cytosol receptors and enzyme induction *in vivo*. *Biochem Biophys Res Commun* 47: 1464–1472

129 Ballard PL, Ballard RA (1972) Glucocorticoid receptors and the role of glucocorticoids in fetal lung development. *Proc Natl Acad Sci USA* 69: 2668

130 Ballard PL, Baxter JD, Higgins SJ, Rousseau GG, Tomkins GM (1974) General presence of glucocorticoid receptors in mammalian tissues. *Endocrinology* 94: 998–1002

131 McEwen BS, Weiss JM, Schwartz LS (1968) Selective retention of corticosterone by limbic structures in rat brain. *Nature* 220: 911–912

132 De Kloet ER, Vreugdenhil E, Oitzl MS, Joëls M (1998) Brain corticosteroid receptor balance in health and disease. *Endocrin Rev* 19: 269–301

133 Krozowski ZS, Funder JW (1983) Renal mineralocorticoid receptors and hippocampal corticosterone-binding species have identical steroid specificity. *Proc Natl Acad Sci USA* 80: 6056–6060

134 Funder JW, Pearce PT, Smith R, Smith AI (1988) Mineralocorticoid action: target tissue speci-

ficity is enzyme, not receptor, mediated. *Science* 242: 583–585

135 Rusvai E, Náray-Fejes-Tóth A (1993) A new isoform of 11β-hydroxysteroid dehydrogenase in aldosterone target cells. *J Biol Chem* 268: 10717–10720

136 Ge R-S, Hardy DO, Catterall JF, Hardy MP (1997) Developmental changes in glucocorticoid receptor and 11β-hydroxysteroid dehydrogenase oxidative and reductive activities in rat Leydig cells. *Endocrinology* 138: 5089–5095

137 Pratt WB, Toft DO (1997) Steroid receptor interactions with heat shock proteins and immunophilin chaperones. *Endocrin Rev* 18: 306–360

138 Gehring U (1993) The structure of glucocorticoid receptors. *J Steroid Biochem Molec Biol* 45: 183–190

139 Wira C, Munck A (1970) Specific glucocorticoid receptors in thymus cells. Localization in the nucleus and extraction of the cortisol-receptor complex. *J Biol Chem* 245: 3436–3438

140 Rousseau GG, Baxter JD, Higgins SJ, Tomkins GM (1973) Steroid-induced nuclear binding of glucocorticoid receptors in intact hepatoma cells. *J Mol Biol* 79: 539–554

141 Wira CR, Munck A (1974) Glucocorticoid-receptor complexes in rat thymus cells. "Cytoplasmic"-nuclear transformations. *J Biol Chem* 249: 5328–5336

142 Wigglesworth VB (1960) Metamorphosis and body form. *The. Harvey Lectures 1958–1959.* Academic Press, New York,

143 Schneiderman HA, Gilbert LI (1959) The chemistry and physiology of insect growth hormones. *In*: D Rudnick (ed.): *Cell, Organism and Milieu.* Ronald Press, New York, 157–187

144 Karlson P (1963) New concepts on the mode of action of hormones. *Perspect Biol Med* 6: 203–214

145 Knox WE, Auerbach VH, Lin ECC (1956) Enzymatic and metabolic adaptations in animals. *Physiol Rev* 36: 164–254

146 Goldstein L, Stella EJ, Knox WE (1962) The effect of hydrocortisone on tyrosine-–ketoglutarate transaminase and tryptophan pyrrolase activities in the isolated, perfused rat liver. *J Biol Chem* 237: 1723–1726

147 Giguère V, Hollenberg SM, Rosenfeld MG, Evans RM (1986) Functional domains of the human glucocorticoid receptor. *Cell* 46: 645–652

148 Evans RM (1988) The steroid and thyroid hormone receptor superfamily. *Science* 240: 889–895

149 Carson-Jurica MA, Schrader WT, O'Malley BW (1990) Steroid receptor family: structure and functions. *Endocrin Rev* 11: 201–220

150 Payvar F, Wrange Ö, Carlstedt-Duke J, Okret S, Gustafsson J-Å, Yamamoto KR (1981) Purified glucocorticoid receptors bind selectively *in vitro* to a cloned DNA fragment whose transcription is regulated by glucocorticoids *in vivo*. *Proc Natl Acad Sci USA* 78: 6628–6632

151 Payvar F, DeFranco D, Firestone GL, Edgar B, Wrange Ö, Okret S, Gustafsson J-Å, Yamamoto KR (1983) Sequence-specific binding of glucocorticoid receptor to MTV DNA at sites within and upstream of the transcribed region. *Cell* 35: 381–392

152 Moras D, Gronemeyer H (1998) The nuclear receptor ligand-binding domain: structure and function. *Curr Opin Cell Biol* 10: 384–391

153 McKenna NJ, Lanz RB, O'Malley BW (1998) Nuclear receptor coregulators: cellular and molecular biology. *Endocrin Rev* 20: 321–344

154 Cole TJ, Blendy JA, Monaghan AP, Krieglstein K, Schmid W, Aguzzi A, Fantuzzi G, Hummler E, Unsicker K, Schütz G (1995) Targeted disruption of the glucocorticoid receptor gene blocks adrenergic chromaffin development and severely retards lung maturation. *Gene Develop* 9: 1608–1625

155 Reichardt HM, Kaestner KH, Tuckermann J, Kretz O, Wessely O, Bock R, Gass P, Schmid W, Herrlich P, Angel P, Schütz G (1998) DNA binding of the glucocorticoid receptor is not essential for survival. *Cell* 93: 531–541

Glucocorticoids
ed. by N.J. Goulding and R.J. Flower
© 2001 Birkhäuser Verlag/Switzerland

The development of synthetic glucocorticoids

Luca Parente

*Department of Pharmaceutical Sciences, University of Salerno, Via Ponte Don Melillo, I-84084
Fisciano (Salerno), Italy*

Introduction

In 1949, a paper by P.S. Hench, E.C. Kendall, C.H. Slocumb and H.F. Polley
published in the *Proceedings of the Staff of the Mayo Clinic*, reported the therapeutic action of the compound E (cortisone) and corticotropin in nine patients
with rheumatoid arthritis. As stated by Munck and Guyre [1], the discovery of
the anti-inflammatory effects of adrenal glucocorticoid hormones "dealt glucocorticoid physiology a blow from which it has yet to recover". On the other
hand, this discovery has flung the door open to the therapy of immuno-inflammatory diseases for the benefit of millions of people. Since these pivotal observations several synthetic glucocorticoids have been synthetized by the pharmaceutical industry and are largely used in a number of inflammatory and
immunologic disorders as potent anti-inflammatory and immunosuppressive
compounds. However, the problem of severe side-effects caused by glucocorticoid treatment has been only partially solved by the newer compounds,
which lack mineralocorticoid activity, but retain the metabolic effects of the
natural hormones. In other words the most potent anti-inflammatory steroids
also produce the most severe side-effects.

Natural steroid hormones

Corticosteroid hormones are synthetized from cholesterol by the adrenal cortex under the control of adrenocorticotropic hormone (ACTH) released by
adenohypophysis. The production of ACTH is in turn controlled by corticotropin-releasing hormone (CRH) released by endocrine hypothalamus (the
hypothalamic-pituitary-adrenal (HPA) axis is discussed in detail in the chapter
of Cowell and Buckingham). The adrenal cortex produces three different types
of hormones: (i) glucocorticoids which regulate carbohydrate, protein and
lipid metabolism; (ii) mineralocorticoids which regulate water and electrolyte
balance; (iii) androgens. The over-all rate of biosynthesis of adrenal steroids is
determined by the rate of supply of cholesterol to the cytochrome P450 local-

ized in the inner layer of the mitochondrial membrane. The cytochrome oxidizes cholesterol to pregnenolone which is the precursor of all steroids. This step is rapidly stimulated by ACTH and is rate-limiting for steroidogenesis. The main glucocorticoid hormone released by the human adrenal cortex is cortisol (hydrocortisone). In the normal adult in the absence of stress, 10–20 mg of cortisol is secreted daily. The rate of secretion follows a circadian rhythm with peak blood concentrations (140–180 ng/ml) in the early morning hours and the lowest concentration (20–40 ng/ml) during the afternoon. Cortisol has widespread and dramatic effects on metabolism of carbohydrates, proteins and lipids (see below). Through these actions cortisol is the main custodian of homeostasis, preserving the normal function of the cardiovascular system, the immune system, the kidney (together with mineralocorticoids like aldosterone), skeletal muscle, the endocrine system, and the nervous system. For many years these physiological effects have been distinguished from pharmacological actions (anti-inflammatory and immunosuppressive) obtainable at higher steroid concentrations. More recently, the observations that both types of effects are mediated by the same glucocorticoid receptor and that the daily production rate of cortisol can rise markedly (at least 10-fold) in stress conditions have wiped out the difference between physiological and pharmacological actions of glucocorticoids. Thus, the various glucocorticoid derivatives used as pharmacological compounds have side-effects on physiological processes that parallel their therapeutic effectiveness.

From natural to synthetic glucocorticoids

After the introduction of *cortisone* (1948) and later *cortisol* (1951) for the treatment of rheumatoid arthritis, many investigators began to search for superior agents having fewer side-effects. Although the natural glucocorticoids can be obtained from animal adrenals, pharmaceutical steroids are usually synthetized from cholic acid or steroid sapogenins that are found in plants of the *Liliaceae* and *Dioscoreaceae* families. Further modifications of these steroids have led to the marketing of a large group of synthetic steroids with special characteristics of relevant pharmacological and therapeutic importance.

The development of synthetic glucocorticoids. Structure-activity relationship

Cortisol (hydrocortisone, Fig. 1), the natural hormone, possesses both glucocorticoid and mineralocorticoid properties as it is able to stimulate both glucocorticoid and mineralocorticoid receptors. Chemical modifications of the cortisol molecule have generated compounds endowed with potent glucocorticoid action, but with negligible effects on water and electrolyte balance since they are ineffective on the mineralocorticoid receptor. On the other hand, since the anti-inflammatory and metabolic effects of glucocorticoids are mediated

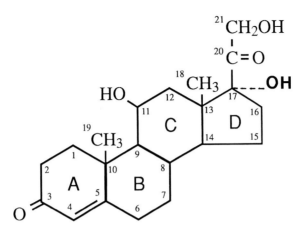

Figure 1. Structure of cortisol (hydrocortisone).

by the same glucocorticoid receptor, the most potent anti-inflammatory steroids also produce profound alterations of carbohydrate, protein, and lipid metabolism as well as a marked suppression of the HPA axis. Changes in molecular structure may bring about changes in biological potency as a result of alterations in absorptions, protein binding, rate of metabolic transformation, rate of excretion, ability to traverse membranes, and intrinsic effectiveness of the molecule at its site of action.

The basic chemical structure of the glucocorticoids is that of cyclopentaneperhydrophenanthrene formed by the three rings (A, B, C) of phenanthrene plus a five-membered cyclopentane ring (D) (Fig. 1). Orientation of the groups attached to the steroid ring system is crucial for biological activity. The groups projecting below the plane of the steroid are designated α, while those projecting above the plane of the molecule are designated β. The essential features for biological activity are the following: (i) a ketone oxygen at C-3 and C-20; (ii) a double bond between C-4 and C-5; (iii) a β-hydroxyl group at C-11; (iv) a 2-carbon chain in β orientation and a hydroxyl group in α at C-17; (v) a β-methyl group at C-18 and C-19. As discussed above the aim of the chemical modifications introduced in the cortisol molecule has been to produce enhanced potency and to separate anti-inflammatory (and, unfortunately, glucocorticoid) action from effects on water and electrolyte balance. Figure 2 shows the structures of commonly used synthetic glucocorticoids.

Chronologically, the first modification performed was the introduction of halogens in the steroid molecule. Fluorination of the cortisol in C-9α, as in *fludrocortisone*, enhances both glucocorticoid and mineralocorticoid activity, apparently by electron-withdrawing effect on the nearby 11β-hydroxyl group. Fludrocortisone (9α-fluorocortisol) has increased glucocorticoid activity (10-fold relative to cortisol), but is even more potent as mineralocorticoid (125-

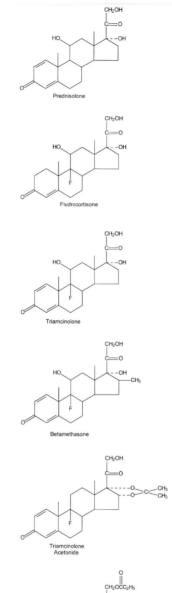

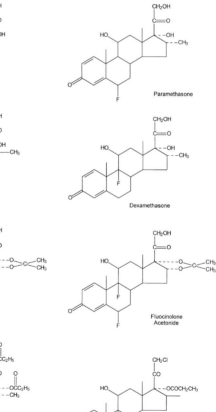

Figure 2. Structures of commonly used synthetic glucocorticoids.

fold relative to cortisol), for this reason it is used in mineralocorticoid replacement therapy. This drug, introduced in 1954, helped to provide the impetus for the synthesis and biologic evaluation of newer halogen-containing analogues.

One year after fludrocortisone, the Δ-corticoids were brought forth into clinical medicine. Investigators at Schering observed that introduction of a double bond between C-1 and C-2 as in *prednisone* and *prednisolone* increased anti-inflammatory activity of about five-fold and reduced mineralo-corticoid effects compared to cortisone and cortisol. In addition, these Δ-corticoids are metabolized more slowly than the natural hormone (Tab. 1). Cortisone and prednisone are 11-keto compounds and lack anti-inflammatory activity until converted into the 11β-hydroxyl compounds, cortisol and prednisolone. The increased potency of the Δ-corticoids may reflect the change in geometry of ring A caused by the introduction of the double bond. Prednisone and prednisolone represent the first chemical innovation leading to modified compounds that could be used in rheumatoid arthritis. When used as anti-rheumatic drugs, smaller doses are required than of cortisol; the usual dose is 5 mg two to four times a day. When equivalent anti-rheumatic doses are given to patients, the Δ-corticoids promote the same pattern of initial improvement as cortisol during the first few months of therapy. The results of longer-term therapy have been significantly better with the modified compounds in terms of efficacy and fewer side-effects. Although these analogs have unwanted side-effects, most clinical investigators prefer the Δ-corticoids to the natural hormones for rheumatoid patients who require steroid therapy. The reasons are that these drugs have less tendency to cause salt and water retention and potassium loss, and that they restore improvement in a significant percentage of patients whose therapeutic control has been lost during cortisone and cortisol therapy. The addition of a methyl group in position C-6α yields *methylprednisolone*, synthetized in 1956, which has slightly greater anti-inflammatory potency and less electrolyte-regulating activity than prednisolone. *Deflazacort*

Table 1. Biological activity, half-life and dosage of some natural and synthetic glucocorticoids

	Anti-inflammatory potency	Mineralo-corticoid potency	Plasma half-life (min)	Biologic half-life (h)	Equivalent oral dose (mg)
Cortisol (hydrocortisone)	1	1	90	8–12	20
Cortisone	0.8	0.8		8–12	25
Prednisolone	4	0.8	200	12–36	5
Prednisone	4	0.8		12–36	5
Methylprednisolone	5	0.5	200	12–36	4
Triamcinolone	5	0	200	12–36	4
Paramethasone	10	0		36–72	2
Betamethasone	25	0	300	36–72	0.75
Desamethasone	25	0	300	36–72	0.75

is a recent oxazoline derivative of prednisolone. Both short- and long-term studies have shown deflazacort to be as effective as prednisone or methylprednisolone in patients with either rheumatoid arthritis or juvenile chronic arthritis. The use of deflazacort appears to be associated with less metabolic side-effects, but further long-term trials are required to confirm this [2].

A natural extension of the corticoid research involved examination of compounds containing both a 9α-fluoro group and a double bond between C-1 and C-2. However, as mentioned previously, the 9α-fluoro group increases both anti-inflammatory and mineralocorticoid potency. By inserting a 16α-hydroxy group into the molecule one can decrease the mineralocorticoid activity. These considerations led to the synthesis in 1958 of *triamcinolone* that shows the same anti-inflammatory potency as methylprednisolone.

Research with 16-methyl substituted corticoids was initiated because investigators hoped to stabilise the 17β-ketol side chain to metabolism. A 16-methyl group is able to increase the stability of the drug in human plasma *in vitro* and the anti-inflammatory activity *in vivo*. Moreover, the methyl group appears to reduce markedly the salt retaining properties of the compound. These studies led, in 1958, to the development of the most potent anti-inflammatory steroids, *dexamethasone* and *betamethasone*. These compounds possess a fluorine atom in position C-9α, which increases glucocorticoid activity, and a methyl group at C-16, which reduces mineralocorticoid activity, in position α for dexamethasone and in position β for betamethasone. These steroids are 25-fold more potent than cortisol as anti-inflammatory compounds and have a longer half-life (Tab. 1). In practical management, 0.75 mg of dexamethasone or betamethasone promotes a therapeutic response equivalent to that from 4 mg of triamcinolone or methylprednisolone, 5 mg of prednisolone, and 20 mg of cortisol. However, since the striking increase in potency correlates to the severity of metabolic side-effects, the therapeutic index of dexamethasone or betamethasone is not higher than that of prednisolone. These potent steroids may be useful when other compounds are no longer effective.

Paramethasone acetate, synthetized in 1960, is a modification of dexamethasone. Paramethasone retains the 16α-methyl group, but the 9α-fluoro group has been moved to the 6α position, in order to reduce the electrolyte loss caused by dexamethasone.

Additional fluorinated analogs like *fluorometholone* or *fluocinolone* are dispensed only for topical administration. Some substitutions have been introduced to obtain lipophilic compounds with high topical anti-inflammatory activity and minimal systemic effects. Examples include the introduction of an acetonide group between hydroxyl groups at C-16 and C-17, as in *triamcinolone acetonide* or *fluocinolone acetonide* (100-fold more potent than cortisol topically), or the esterification of the C-17 hydroxyl group with valerate or benzoate, as in some betamethasone derivatives.

Newer synthetic derivatives have incorporated chlorine atoms into the steroid molecule. *Beclomethasone*, a 9α-chloro analog of betamethasone, is a potent glucocorticoid, and the dipropionate derivative is utilised in inhalation therapy for asthma. Substitution of the hydroxyl group at C-21 with chlorine, as in *clobetasol propionate*, provides high topical anti-inflammatory activity.

Recent derivatives used as anti-inflammatory drugs following local application are *budesonide, mometasone furoate* and *fluticasone propionate*. These drugs are both highly lipophilic and rapidly inactivated following absorption. Hepatic first-pass metabolism inactivates about 80% of these drugs, but only 20% of the systemic glucocorticoids, thus minimizing their systemic side-effects. In a recent clinical study, budesonide has been compared to prednisolone in the local treatment of active Crohn's disease. Treatment with budesonide was nearly as effective as prednisolone and associated with fewer side-effects and less suppression of pituitary-adrenal function [3]. More recently, several commonly used inhaled glucocorticoids were tested for their ability to inhibit expression of either vascular cell adhesion molecule-1 (VCAM-1) and intercellular adhesion molecule-1 (ICAM-1). All glucocorticoids tested inhibited VCAM-1 expression in a dose-dependent manner. No inhibition of ICAM-1 was observed. The most potent drugs in inhibiting VCAM-1 expression were mometasone furoate and fluticasone propionate. Budesonide, triamcinolone acetonide, and beclomethasone dipropionate had intermediate potency, while cortisol was the least potent of the steroids tested [4].

Novel experimental synthetic analogs

One original and interesting approach toward development of locally active anti-inflammatory steroids is based upon the concept of antedrug developed by a group working at Florida A&M University. The term antedrug is used to describe an active compound synthetized by chemically modifying an active parent compound to enhance its local activity. The new compound is designed to be rapidly metabolized to inactive compounds upon entry into the systemic circulation from the tissue to which it was applied. On this basis a number of prednisolone derivatives have been synthetized and tested for their pharmacological properties.

A series of 16α-alkoxycarbonyl-17-deoxyprednisolone derivatives has been synthetized and tested locally in both the acute croton oil-induced ear edema and the cotton pellet granuloma in the rat. The analogs showed an increased local anti-inflammatory activity compared to prednisolone. As expected, prednisolone caused significant side-effects, such as reduction in thymus weights, body weight increase, and suppression of plasma corticosterone levels. Unlike prednisolone, the novel analogs had virtually no impact on the above parameters of systemic effects compared to control values [5]. Similar results have been obtained with different analogs, the 9α-fluoro-16-methoxycarbonylprednisolone and its 21-acetate derivative. These compounds also exhibit an increased topical anti-inflammatory activity, compared to that of prednisolone, without significant adverse systemic effects [6, 7]. These promising results ought to be confirmed in a clinical setting.

Pharmacokinetics

The gastro-intestinal tract effectively absorbs cortisol and synthetic derivatives. The introduction of phosphate or hemisuccinate groups at C-21 increases the water solubility and allows the parenteral administration of these drugs. Glucocorticoids are also absorbed from sites of local application such as synovial spaces, the conjunctival sac, and the skin. When administration is prolonged or when large areas of the skin are involved, the absorption may lead to systemic side-effects.

In plasma, cortisol and synthetic derivatives are reversibly bound to a specific transport globulin, transcortin, and to albumin. Transcortin is a globulin with high affinity and low total binding capacity, while albumin has low affinity, but relatively large binding capacity. At low or normal concentrations, 80–90% of both cortisol and prednisolone are bound to transcortin and only 5–10% are bound to albumin. At higher concentrations, transcortin-binding sites become saturated, resulting in an increase of free cortisol and prednisolone that can be metabolized. Thus, the rate of elimination of cortisol and prednisolone increases at higher dosing regimens. Conversely, as methylprednisolone and dexamethasone are essentially bound only to albumin, the percentage of binding is concentration independent. Thus, the rate of elimination of both methylprednisolone and dexamethasone remains constant regardless of dose.

Glucocorticoids are generally metabolized through reduction of the double bond between C-4 and C-5, which can occur at both hepatic and extrahepatic sites, followed by reduction of the ketone group in C-3 to a hydroxyl group, which has been demonstrated only in the liver. Most of the reduced, inactive metabolites are enzymatically coupled through the C-3 hydroxyl with sulfate or with glucuronic acid to yield water-soluble sulfate esters or glucuronides, which are excreted as such by the kidney. Half-life time values show that the presence of a double bond between C-1 and C-2 (prednisolone, methylprednisolone) and of a fluorine at C-6 (paramethasone), or at C-9 (betamethasone, dexamethasone) increases the resistance of the molecules to degradation and reduces their clearance so that these drugs are able to exert prolonged effects in the body (Tab. 1).

The mechanism of action of glucocorticoids

Glucocorticoids interact with specific cytosolic receptors to regulate the expression of responsive genes, thereby either up-regulating or down-regulating the synthesis of specific proteins by the various target tissues. These receptors, about 3000 to 10 000 per cell, belong to a superfamily of nuclear receptors stimulated by other small hydrophobic ligands like mineralocorticoids, sex steroids, thyroid hormones, vitamin D, and retinoids. The glucocorticoid receptor is a 777-aminoacid protein that functions, when stimulated, as transcription factor. The inactivated receptors are localized in the cytoplasm anchored to inhibitory proteins of the HSP family. The steroid ligand diffuses across the membrane of the target cells and interacts with the steroid-binding domain at the carboxy terminus of the receptor. The inhibitory protein(s) dissociates from the receptor, which undergoes a conformational change that exposes the DNA-binding domain formed by two "zinc fingers" where a zinc ion binds to a pair of cysteines and a pair of histidines. The complex ligand-receptor dimerizes and translocates to the nucleus where the zinc fingers bind to specific DNA sequences known as glucocorticoid-responsive elements (GRE) in the promoter region of responsive genes. Two types of GRE are known, the positive and the negative GRE, which stimulate and inhibit gene expression respectively (for further details see the chapters of Oakley and Cidlowski). The activated dimer can also interfere with the function of other transcription factors. It is known that the complex can inhibit the transactivating activity of factors like AP-1 (a heterodimer of Fos and Jun proteins) [8] and NF-κB [9] by direct physical association with these factors, thereby sequestering them from their binding sites on DNA sequences.

Recently, a different mechanism of inhibition of NF-κB activity has been elucidated. In unstimulated cells NF-κB is localized in the cytoplasm complexed with inhibitory proteins IκBα and IκBβ. When cells are stimulated, specific kinases phosphorylate the suppressor molecules, promoting their degradation by proteasomes. The release of NF-κB from IκB causes the translocation of NF-κB into the nucleus, where it binds to specific sequences in the promoter regions of target genes. It has been shown that glucocorticoids induce the transcription of the gene encoding IκBα. The increase in IκBα mRNA results in increased synthesis IκBα protein which traps activated NF-κB in inactive cytoplasmic complexes [10, 11]. However, different reports have shown that this is not a general mechanism, suggesting that the increased synthesis of IκBα is not sufficient for the steroid-mediated down-modulation of NF-κB activity [12, 13].

A recent study has investigated the ability of various glucocorticoids to induce gene expression and apoptosis and to repress NF-κB-dependent transcription [13]. The ability to induce gene expression and apoptosis paralleled the anti-inflammatory potency. In fact, clobetasol, dexamethasone, betamethasone and triamcinolone turned out to be the best inducers of both gene expression and apoptosis while prednisolone and cortisol caused a low to intermediate degree of induction. On the other hand, the NF-κB activation induced by TNF-α was significantly reduced by all glucocorticoids to a comparable extent. In these experiments no increase in expression of IκBα was detected, suggesting that the inhibition of NF-κB activity was due to mechanisms involving protein-protein interaction rather than induction of IκBα.

The interaction with the glucocorticoid receptor accounts for most of the metabolic actions of natural and synthetic glucocorticoids as well as for their anti-inflammatory and immunosuppressive properties. One possible way to separate beneficial from deleterious effect is to dissociate transactivation from transrepression inasmuch as gene repression may be responsible for the immunosuppressive and anti-inflammatory effects while several metabolic effects may be due to gene activation. A recent paper has addressed this issue [14]. Some analogs, termed "dissociated glucocorticoids" have been identified which efficiently transrepress AP-1 activity, while only marginally activating steroid-responsive genes. These analogs inhibit the release of IL-1 from cultured cells and show *in vivo* anti-inflammatory activity comparable to that of classical glucocorticoids such as dexamethasone and prednisolone. It is not yet known if these analogs have fewer side-effects than classical glucocorticoids.

Recently, nongenomic glucocorticoid actions not mediated by cytosolic receptors have been described. These effects which are caused by high dose glucocorticoids may be mediated by either membrane receptors or by physicochemical interactions with cellular membranes [15]. While these nongenomic mechanisms may well explain rapid onset effects by glucocorticoids like feedback inhibition of ACTH release, further experimental and clinical data are needed to fully elucidate the connection between nongenomic mechanisms and anti-inflammatory effects.

Anti-inflammatory and immunosuppressive effects of glucocorticoids

Through the modulation of gene expression, natural and synthetic glucocorticoids exert their potent anti-inflammatory and immunosuppressive action. Thus, glucocorticoids are able to inhibit the synthesis of pro-inflammatory proteins as well as to induce *de novo* synthesis of anti-inflammatory proteins. The production of most inflammatory cytokines, such as IL-1, IL-2, IL-6, TNFα, interferon-γ, chemokines, like IL-8, adhesion molecules is markedly inhibited by glucocorticoids. The expression of inducible enzymes like cyclooxygenase-2 and nitric oxide synthase as well as the expression of other enzymes involved in inflammatory responses like phospholipase A_2 and collagenase are also reduced by steroid compounds. These inhibitory actions are brought about either by the interaction of the activated glucocorticoid receptor with negative GRE in the promoter regions of responsive genes or by the interference of the receptor with the transactivating properties of transcription factors like AP-1 and NF-κB as discussed above. It is well known that these factors regulate the expression of genes that encode many cytokines, adhesion molecules, and enzymes [16].

A specular facet of the anti-inflammatory activity of glucocorticoids is represented, as mentioned above, by the up-regulation of the synthesis of anti-inflammatory proteins like lipocortin (annexin)-1. It is noteworthy that the potency of synthetic glucocorticoids in inducing the synthesis of lipocortin-1 in cell cultures reflects their anti-inflammatory activity *in vivo* [17]. The anti-inflammatory effects of lipocortin-1 relate to the properties of the protein to inhibit both phospholipase A_2 activity [18] and neutrophil activation and migration ([19], see also the chapters by Pitzalis et al. and Cowell). The capability of glucocorticoids to induce lipocortin-1 has been differently reported inasmuch as the steroid induction is dependent on tissues examined, state of cell differentiation and possibly additional factors ([20] and references therein). Recently, it has been shown that the promoter of lipocortin-1 can be considered a slow responder to steroid treatment and that protein induction is a secondary glucocorticoid response requiring new protein synthesis [21].

Side-effects of natural and synthetic glucocorticoids

In general, the side-effects of glucocorticoids are common to all such agents. There does not appear to be any complication of glucocorticoid therapy unique to a particular agent. Two categories of toxic effects result from the therapeutic use of glucocorticoids: those resulting from prolonged use of pharmacological doses and those resulting from withdrawal of therapy. These effects are characteristic of the iatrogenic Cushing's syndrome that is present, with a different degree of severity and clinical signs, in all patients receiving pharmacological doses of glucocorticoids for more than 2–3 weeks. Short-term therapy, even with high doses, is not usually accompanied by serious consequences.

For clinical purposes glucocorticoid side-effects can be distinguished in common effects related to dose and duration of therapy and sporadic effects not directly related to dose and duration of treatment (Tab. 2). The dose-related effects are generally predictable from the actions of glucocorticoids on intermediary metabolism and on the different tissues and organs described in the following paragraphs. Besides dose and duration of therapy, patient factors

Table 2. Toxicity of glucocorticoid therapy

Dose-related effects
- Sodium retention, hypokalemia (only natural hormones)
- HPA axis suppression
- Glucose intolerance, hyperglycemia
- Redistribution of body fat with truncal obesity
- Osteoporosis
- Skin fragility with petechiae and ecchymoses
- Impaired wound healing
- Immunosuppression with susceptibilty to opportunistic infections
- Growth retardation
- Myopathy

Dose-unrelated effects
- Mood alterations, psychosis
- Benign intracranial hypertension
- Cataracts and glaucoma
- Peptic ulcer
- Hypertension
- Aseptic necrosis of femoral and humeral heads
- Acute pancreatitis
- Anaphylactoid reactions

must be taken into account in order to establish a correct glucocorticoid treatment. Elderly patients tend to have an increased incidence of side-effects
whenever they are affected by conditions such as glucose intolerance, muscle
weakness or osteoporosis, which may be worsened by glucocorticoids.
Chronically ill or malnourished individuals may tolerate steroids poorly
because of decreased concentration of serum proteins and a related increase in
levels of active, unbound drug. The dose-unrelated effects are often of
unknown origin and affect a limited number of treated patients either early or
late during the course of therapy.

Effects of natural and synthetic glucocorticoids on metabolism

Carbohydrate and protein metabolism

The profound effects of natural and synthetic glucocorticoids on carbohydrate
and protein metabolism tend to increase blood glucose levels. Thus, treatment
with glucocorticoids can worsen control in patients with overt diabetes and can
precipitate hyperglycemia in predisposed individuals. On the other hand, the
physiological function of these effects is to protect glucose-dependent tissues,
such as the brain and heart, from starvation. In the liver, glucocorticoids promote both the formation of glucose from amino acids and glycerol and the
storage of glucose as glycogen. In peripheral tissues, especially muscle, glucocorticoids act to decrease the utilization of glucose and to mobilise amino
acids from the breakdown of proteins. Amino acids are then carried to the liver,
where they form the substrate for gluconeogenesis. Several mechanisms are
involved in these effects. Glucocorticoids induce the transcription of a number
of hepatic enzymes involved in gluconeogenesis and amino acid metabolism,
including phosphoenolpyruvate carboxykinase, glucose-6-phosphatase, and
fructose-2,6-biphosphatase. Glucocorticoids inhibit peripheral glucose uptake
by reducing the number of glucose carrier molecules on the membrane of
adipocytes and skeletal muscle cells.

Lipid metabolism

Both natural and synthetic glucocorticoids promote a dramatic redistribution
of body fat with increased fat deposition in the back of the neck (*buffalo
hump*), face (*moon face*), and supraclavicular area, and a loss of fat in the
extremities. Moreover, glucocorticoids facilitate the lipolytic action of other
agents, such as growth hormone and β-adrenergic receptor agonists. It has
been proposed that body fat redistribution is caused by different sensitivities of
peripheral and truncal adipocytes to the lipogenic action of insulin, produced
in response to the hyperglycemia, *versus* the glucocorticoid-facilitated lipolytic effects.

Salt and water metabolism

Aldosterone, the main mineralocorticoid hormone secreted by the adrenals, acts *via* the mineralocorticoid receptor to regulate water and electrolyte balance. Cortisol, the natural glucocorticoid hormone, is also able to interact with the mineralocorticoid receptor promoting water and sodium retention as well as urinary excretion of potassium and hydrogen ions. These effects cause expansion of the extracellular fluid volume, slight increase in plasma sodium concentration, hypokalemia, and alkalosis. Recent synthetic derivatives do not interact with mineralocorticoid receptors and are devoid of such effects on electrolyte balance.

Calcium metabolism

Natural and synthetic glucocorticoids inhibit intestinal absorption of calcium by down-regulating the synthesis of an intestinal calcium binding protein causing secondary hyperparathyroidism. Parathyroid hormone, in turn, stimulates osteoclasts to increase bone resorption. In addition, steroid drugs directly inhibit the activity of osteoblasts and stimulate the urinary excretion of both calcium and phosphorus. All these effects contribute to severe osteoporosis that may represent an indication for withdrawal of therapy.

Effects of natural and synthetic glucocorticoids on different tissues and organs

Hypothalamus-pituitary-adrenal (HPA) axis

Glucocorticoids suppress endogenous secretion of both ACTH and cortisol. The degree and duration of HPA suppression and, consequently, the amount of time required for recovery of function depend on dose and duration of therapy. In general, the suspicion of an initial HPA suppression should arise in any patient who has received the equivalent to 20–30 mg of prednisone per day for more than a week. Since it is difficult to predict the time required for recovery after a few weeks of therapy, HPA suppression should be suspected for 12 months after such a course of treatment. The most severe complication of steroid withdrawal is acute adrenal insufficiency caused by abrupt cessation of therapy. This life-threatening disease is characterised by gastrointestinal symptoms, dehydration, hyponatremia, hyperkalemia, weakness, lethargy, and hypotension.

In addition to this most severe form of withdrawal, a characteristic steroid withdrawal syndrome consists of anorexia, fever, myalgia, arthralgia, nausea, malaise, and postural hypotension. Many of these symptoms occur in patients with both normal plasma cortisol levels and normal HPA function. Thus, this type of withdrawal syndrome does not depend on low cortisol levels or the impairment of HPA responsiveness. As previously discussed, glucocorticoids inhibit the synthesis and release of both IL-1 and prostaglandins, mediators able to produce many of the signs of the withdrawal syndrome. Therefore, it has been proposed that this syndrome be caused by a sudden increase in IL-1 and prostaglandin formation following the withdrawal of exogenous glucocorticoids.

A recent double-blind, randomized, placebo-controlled study has compared the effects on HPA axis of fluticasone propionate aerosol, triamcinolone acetonide aerosol, prednisone, and placebo. After 4 weeks of treatment the adrenal response to cosyntropin infusion was evaluated. The mean plasma cortisol response to cosyntropin was similar among fluticasone, triamcinolone and placebo groups, while it was significantly reduced after treatment with prednisone [22]. These results indicate that newer synthetic steroid analogs may be less toxic for the HPA axis compared to traditional compounds.

Blood leukocytes

The administration of glucocorticoids causes a decrease in circulating eosinophils, lymphocytes, and monocytes. This appears to be due to cell redistribution into extravascular compartments as well as to steroid-induced apoptosis of both eosinophils and lymphocytes. Conversely, the number of circulating neutrophils is increased by glucocorticoids. Both a diminished adherence of neutrophils to endothelial cells and an acute release of neutrophils from the bone marrow bring about this increase. The net result is that fewer cells are available at the site of tissue injury to mediate host response. These actions together with the potent immunosuppressive effects of glucocorticoids on cytokines, discussed above, may lead to an increased susceptibility to opportunistic infection such as *Pneumocystitis carinii* pneumonia, or cryptococcal meningitis, or reactivation of latent tuberculosis.

Central nervous system

Natural glucocorticoid hormones have important homeostatic effects on the brain by regulating blood glucose levels and electrolyte balance. On the other hand, therapeutic administration of these drugs may cause an array of neurological signs ranging from slight mood changes to schizophrenic psychoses. The molecular mechanisms of these effects are unknown, but may involve $GABA_A$ receptors. Locally produced steroids, termed "neurosteroids", activate these receptors to regulate neuronal excitability.

Cardiovascular system

Both natural and synthetic glucocorticoids tend to increase blood pressure through different mechanisms: sodium and water retention (only natural hormones), vasoconstriction, increased myocardial contractility. Vasoconstriction may be caused by inhibition of the synthesis of vasodilator mediators like prostacyclin and nitric oxide and also by permissive effects on the vasoconstrictor action of catecolamines and angiotensin II. These permissive effects as well as the increase of myocardial contractility may be mediated by steroid-induced up-regulation of the number and affinity of adrenergic receptors due to promoter sites on the receptor genes.

Gastrointestinal system

The risk of developing peptic ulcers during glucocorticoid therapy has been differently reported. The use of glucocorticoids may worsen a pre-existent peptic ulcer or potentiate the gastric mucosa damaging effects of non-steroidal anti-inflammatory drugs.

Connective tissue

High doses of natural and synthetic glucocorticoids inhibit the formation of both collagen (type I and type III) and glycosaminoglycan by fibroblasts. Biosynthesis of type I collagen involves transcription of two different procollagen genes, pro-A1 and pro-A2, and translation of mRNAs into the corresponding prepro-A-collagen proteins. The cellular accumulation of the mRNAs is reduced by glucocorticoids. This is not due to a decrease in gene transcription, but to an increase in the rate of degradation of the specific mRNAs possibly mediated by a steroid-induced increase in ribonuclease activity. These effects lead to the characteristic thinning and fragility of the skin as well as to the delayed wound healing observed in the iatrogenic Cushing's syndrome. The inhibitory effects on connective tissues are in part responsible for the growth retardation caused by glucocorticoids in children. In addition, glucocorticoids block the action of somatomedin C in promoting linear growth.

Skeletal muscle

Excessive amounts of glucocorticoids, either from high dose therapy or endogenous hypercorticism, impair muscle function. Steroid drugs promote skeletal muscle wasting *via* unknown mechanisms. This steroid-induced myopathy may be an indication for withdrawal of therapy.

Eye

Glucocorticoids tend to increase intraocular pressure, leading in some cases to posterior subcapsular cataracts. The mechanisms may involve both increased production of aqueous humor and reduced drainage. A pre-existent glaucoma represents a contraindication for steroid therapy.

Conclusions and perspectives

Synthetic glucocorticoids are the mainstay in the therapy of many serious immuno-inflammatory diseases. Their prolonged use may ameliorate dramatically the quality of life of patients, but is often associated with life-threatening toxicity. Several lines of investigation, outlined in the previous paragraphs, aim to the development of safer steroid-like drugs. Examples are site-specific glucocorticoid derivatives for local inflammatory disorders, such as asthma and skin diseases. Newer drugs, already in the clinic, and experimental compounds, like steroid antedrugs, are potent local anti-inflammatory agents with minimal systemic side-effects. Research on dissociated glucocorticoids as well as on lipocortin-derived peptides may lead to compounds with fewer metabolic effects. Finally, it is important to realize that many of the clinical uses of glucocorticoids are based on empirical approaches, with the exception of replacement therapy in HPA axis deficiency states. Therefore, more basic research is needed, aimed at a better understanding of both the pathology of immuno-inflammatory disorders and the intimate molecular mechanisms of glucocorticoid action.

References

1 Munck A, Guyre PM (1989) Glucocorticoid physiology and homeostasis in relation to anti-inflammatory actions. *In*: RP Schleimer, HN Claman, A Oronsky (eds): *Anti-inflammatory steroid action. Basic and clinical aspects.* Academic Press, San Diego, 30–47
2 Markham A, Bryson HM (1995) Deflazacort. A review of its pharmacological properties and therapeutic efficacy. *Drugs* 50: 317–333
3 Rutgeerts P, Löfberg R, Malchow H, Lamers C, Olaison G, Jewell D, Danielsson Å, Goebell H, Thomsen OØ, Lorenz-Meyer H et al (1994) A comparison of budesonide with prednisolone for active Crohn's disease. *N Engl J Med* 331: 842–845
4 Atsuta J, Plitt J, Bochner BS, Schleimer RP (1999) Inhibition of VCAM-1 expression in human bronchial cells by glucocorticoids. *Amer J Respir Cell Mol Biol* 20: 643–650
5 Yoon K-J, Khalil MA, Kwon T, Choi S-J, Lee HJ (1995) Steroidal anti-inflammatory antedrugs: synthesis and pharmacological evaluation of 16α-alkoxycarbonyl-17-deoxyprednisolone derivatives. *Steroids* 60: 445–451
6 Heiman AS, Ko D-H, Chen M, Lee HJ (1997) New steroidal anti-inflammatory antedrugs: methyl 3,20-dioxo-9α-fluoro-11β,17α,21-trihydroxy-1,4-pregnadiene-16α–carboxylate and methyl 21-acetyloxy-3,20-dioxo-11β,17α–dihydroxy-9α–fluoro-1,4-pregnadiene-16α carboxylate. *Steroids* 62: 491–499
7 Heiman AS, Hickman F, Ko D-H, Lee HJ (1998) New steroidal anti-inflammatory antedrugs bind to macrophage glucocorticoid receptors and inhibit nitric oxide generation. *Steroids* 63: 644–649

8 Jonat C, Rahmsdorf HJ, Park KK, Cato AC, Gebel S, Ponta H, Herrlich P (1990) Antitumor promotion and antiinflammation: down-modulation of AP-1 (Fos/Jun) activity by glucocorticoid hormone. *Cell* 62: 1189–1204

9 Ray A, Prefontaine KE (1994) Physical association and functional antagonism between the p65 subunit of transcription factor NF-κB and the glucocorticoid receptor. *Proc Natl Acad Sci USA* 91: 752–756

10 Scheinman RI, Cogswell PC, Lofquist AK, Baldwin ASJ (1995) Role of transcriptional activation of IκBα in mediation of immunosuppression by glucocorticoids. *Science* 270: 283–286

11 Auphan N, DiDonato JA, Rosette C, Helmberg A, Karin M (1995) Immunosuppression by glucocorticoids: inhibition of NF-κB activity through induction of IκB synthesis. *Science* 270: 286–290

12 Heck S, Bender K, Kullmann M, Gottlicher M, Herrlich P, Cato ACB (1997) IκBα-independent downregulation of NF-κB activity by glucocorticoid receptor. *EMBO J* 16: 4698–4707

13 Hofmann TG, Hehner SP, Bacher S, Droge W, Schmitz ML (1998) Various glucocorticoids differ in their ability to induce gene expression, apoptosis and to repress NF-κB-dependent transcription. *FEBS Lett* 441: 441–446

14 Vayssiere BM, Dupont S, Choquart A, Petit F, Garcia T, Marchandeau C, Gronemeyer H, Resche-Rigon M (1997) Synthetic glucocorticoids that dissociate transactivation and AP-1 transrepression exhibit antiinflammatory activity *in vivo*. *Mol Endocrinol* 11: 1245–1255

15 Buttgereit F, Wehling M, Burmester G-R (1998) A new hypothesis of modular glucocorticoid actions. *Arthritis Rheum* 41: 761–767

16 Barnes PJ, Karin M (1997) Nuclear factor-κB. A pivotal transcription factor in chronic inflammatory diseases. *N Engl J Med* 336: 1066–1071

17 Blackwell GJ, Parente L (1985) Macrocortin, a glucocorticoid-induced regulator of cell function. *Lymphokines* 11: 187–211

18 Flower RJ, Rothwell NJ (1994) Lipocortin-1: cellular mechanisms and clinical relevance. *Trends Pharmacol* 15: 71–76

19 Perretti M, Croxtall JD, Wheller SK, Goulding NJ, Hannon R, Flower RJ (1996) Mobilizing lipocortin 1 in adherent human leukocytes downregulates their transmigration. *Nat Med* 2: 1259–1262

20 Parente L, Solito E (1994) Association between glucocorticosteroids and lipocortin 1. *Trends Pharmacol* 15: 362

21 Solito E, de Coupade C, Parente L, Flower RJ, Russo-Marie F (1998) Human annexin 1 is highly expressed during the differentiation of the epithelial cell line A 549: involvement of nuclear factor interleukin 6 in phorbol ester induction of annexin 1. *Cell Growth Differ* 9: 327–336

22 Li JT, Goldstein MF, Gross GN, Noonan MJ, Weisberg S, Edwards L, Reed KD, Rogenes PR (1999) Effects of fluticasone propionate, triamcinolone acetonide, prednisone, and placebo on the hypothalamic-pituitary-adrenal axis. *J Allergy Clin Immunol* 103: 622–629

Molecular mechanisms of glucocorticoid action

The glucocorticoid receptor: expression, function, and regulation of glucocorticoid responsiveness

Robert H. Oakley and John A. Cidlowski

Laboratory of Signal Transduction, National Institute of Environmental Health Sciences, National Institutes of Health, Research Triangle Park, North Carolina 27709, USA

Introduction

Glucocorticoids and their synthetic derivatives are among the most widely pre-scribed class of drug in the world today. The ability of both natural and syn-thetic glucocorticoids to act on target tissues and elicit specific biological responses is dependent on the presence of the alpha isoform of the glucocorti-coid receptor (GRα). GRα belongs to the superfamily of steroid/thyroid/retinoic acid receptor proteins that function as ligand-depend-ent transcription factors [1]. Following high affinity binding of the glucocorti-coid hormone, GRα activates or represses transcription of target genes and consequently changes cellular phenotype.

Sensitivity to glucocorticoids varies within the normal population and among patients with different diseases [2]. Certain individuals develop serious side-effects from a low dose of exogenous glucocorticoids, whereas others do not develop side-effects even with a much higher dose administered over a long period of time. In addition, the beneficial effects of glucocorticoids in the treat-ment of many immune and inflammatory diseases is often limited by the devel-opment of resistance in the diseased tissue [3]. Glucocorticoid sensitivity with-in the body varies among tissues and even within the same tissue during dif-ferent stages of development [4]. Changes in cellular sensitivity to glucocorti-coids also occur during the cell cycle [5]. The molecular basis for these varia-tions in glucocorticoid responsiveness, however, is poorly understood [6, 7].

GRα, as the primary effector molecule in the glucocorticoid signaling cas-cade, is the principal target for regulatory events that modulate target cell sen-sitivity to glucocorticoids. Many studies have shown that there is a direct cor-relation between the number of GRα molecules in a cell and the cell's ability to respond to glucocorticoids. Cellular responsiveness to glucocorticoids is also influenced by the potency with which GRα functions as a ligand-depend-ent transcription factor. The profound influence that glucocorticoids have on normal physiology, their extensive use in the treatment of pathological condi-tions, and the development of glucocorticoid resistant states in both normal and diseased tissues necessitate a thorough understanding of the factors that control cellular sensitivity to glucocorticoids by regulating the expression and/or function of GRα. This review begins by discussing the expression pathway for the GR gene and the function of the GRα protein. The remainder of the chapter examines the factors known to regulate the expression of GRα and/or the efficacy with which GRα functions as a ligand-dependent transcription factor. It is the interplay among these factors that ultimately appears to govern target cell sensitivity to glucocorticoids.

Expression pathway of the GR gene and function of GRα

The physiological actions of glucocorticoids are mediated by GRα which converts the endocrine signal into changes in cellular phenotype. Consistent with the widespread actions of glucocorticoids, GRα is expressed in almost all human cells and tissues [8]. GRα is a member of a very large family of ligand-activated transcription factors that includes receptors for the steroid hormones (progesterone, androgen, mineralocorticoid, and estrogen), thyroid hormone, retinoic acid, and vitamin D [1, 9]. This family also includes a large and growing group of proteins termed orphan receptors whose ligand and/or function remains to be identified. Like other members of this superfamily, GRα is comprised of a poorly conserved amino-terminal domain that is involved in gene activation, a highly conserved central DNA binding domain, and a relatively well-conserved carboxy-terminal domain that is important for hormone binding. The expression pathway for the GR gene and the function of the GRα protein in the glucocorticoid signal transduction pathway are discussed in the following section.

Expression pathway of the GR gene

Organization of the GR gene
GRα was one of the first transcription factors cloned from mammalian cells as human, rat, and mouse receptor cDNAs were isolated in rapid succession in the mid 1980s [10–12]. The genomic organization of the GR gene was determined several years later. The human GR gene was initially reported to consist of 10 exons [13]. It was later demonstrated, however, that the last two exons (exon 9α and exon 9β) and the intervening sequences between them (intron J) actually form one large terminal exon [14]. Therefore, as shown in Figure 1A, the human GR gene is comprised of nine exons. The mouse GR gene also consists of 9 exons and is organized in an identical fashion [15]. For both the human and mouse GR genes which are located on chromosome 5, exon 2 contains the translation start site and encodes the amino-terminal portion of the receptor; exons 3 and 4 encode the two zinc fingers of the DNA binding domain (DBD); and the last five exons encode the hormone binding domain

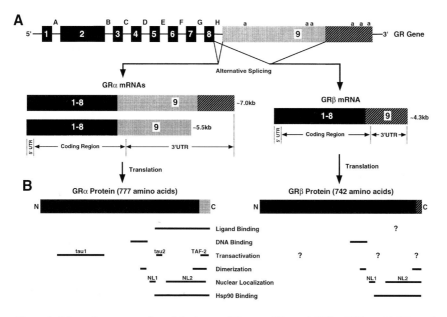

Figure 1. Schematic representation of the human GR gene, GRα and GRβ mRNAs, and GRα and GRβ proteins. A, the human GR gene is comprised of nine exons, and alternative processing of the GR primary transcript produces multiple messages. The normal splicing pathway, which links the end of exon 8 to the beginning of exon 9, generates GRα mRNA transcripts, which differ in size due to alternative polyadenylation (consensus polyadenylation signals located in exon 9 are indicated with a lower case "a"). The alternative splicing pathway, which links the end of exon 8 to downstream sequences in exon 9, generates the GRβ mRNA transcript. B, the GRα and GRβ proteins are identical through amino acid 727, but then diverge. The functional domains and subdomains so far described for each protein are indicated.

(HBD). Exon 1 and the first part of exon 2 contain 5' untranslated region (5'UTR) and exon 9 contains a very large 3' untranslated region (3'UTR).

The promoter of the human GR gene (three kilobases of which has been sequenced) has several features in common with "TATA-less promoters." It lacks typical TATA and CAAT boxes, is GC rich with multiple GC-box consensus sequences (the recognition site for the transcription factor SP-1), and contains multiple transcription start sites [13, 16, 17]. The preponderance of GC-boxes suggests that the promoter is constitutively active [18]. Interestingly, expression of the mouse GR gene is controlled by three different promoters (1A, 1B, and 1C), each of which directs the splicing of a different first exon onto the common exon 2 [15]. The human GR promoter that has been characterized so far corresponds in position and sequence to promoter 1C of the mouse GR gene. Regulation of the GR gene at the level of transcription and the potential significance of the three mouse GR promoters are discussed below.

GRα and GRβ mRNA transcripts

Transcription of the GR gene produces multiple GRα mRNA transcripts (Fig. 1A). The two predominant messages observed on Northern blots of human, rat, and mouse tissues are 7.0 and 5.5 kb in size and originate from alternative polyadenylation in the 3'UTR of exon 9 [14]. The 7.0 kb message contains the full-length 3'UTR (approximately 4.0 kb), and the 5.5 kb message contains approximately 2.4 kb of 3'UTR. These two GRα mRNA transcripts have a widespread tissue distribution, but their relative ratio varies in a tissue-specific manner. In all cases, the 7.0 kb message appears to be more abundant than the 5.5 kb transcript. GRα mRNA heterogeneity also results from alternative splicing. As mentioned above, three different first exons are alternatively spliced onto a common exon 2 to generate mouse GRα mRNA transcripts with different 5'UTRs [15]. Similar observations have been reported in rat, but not in humans [19]. Alternative splicing of the human GR primary transcript produces a splice variant that encodes a receptor protein (GRβ) that differs from the wild-type receptor (GRα) only at the carboxy terminus [14] (Fig. 1, A and B). In the normal splicing pathway, the end of exon 8 is linked to the beginning of exon 9, thus generating the 7.0 and 5.5 kb GRα mRNA transcripts. The alternative splicing event links the end of exon 8 to downstream sequences in exon 9 resulting in the GRβ mRNA transcript. This transcript is approximately 4.3 kb in size and has been detected in many different tissues and cell lines [14, 20]. Semiquantitative RT-PCR analysis of whole tissues indicates that the GRβ message is expressed at significantly lower levels than the GRα mRNA transcripts [14]. However, these results may not reflect the situation in many individual cells since GRβ is expressed in a cell-type specific pattern within tissues [21]. The GRβ-specific sequences are highly conserved in rat and mouse but a rodent homologue of the GRβ transcript has not yet been detected [22].

GRα and GRβ proteins

The GRα protein has been shown by both Western blotting and hormone binding assays to be expressed in almost all cells and tissues, and this ubiquitous expression is consistent with the wide-ranging and diverse set of actions mediated by glucocorticoid hormones. GRα is comprised of 777 amino acids in humans, 795 amino acids in rats, and 783 amino acids in mice [10–12]. These proteins are highly homologous and even identical over large stretches of the polypeptide. The larger size of rat and mouse receptor is due to the presence of a polyglutamine stretch, the significance of which is unknown, in the amino terminal portion of the receptor. The domain structure of human GRα is shown in Figure 1B. The primary transactivation domain (tau 1) resides within the amino-terminal half of the receptor, the DBD is in the middle of the molecule, and the HBD is located in the carboxy-terminal half of the receptor. Separating these three domains are "hinge" regions which are accessible to proteases even when the receptor is in its native conformation. GRα also contains a number of important subdomains involved in transactivation, dimerization, nuclear localization, and binding heat shock protein hsp90 (Fig. 1B). The structure and function of these domains and subdomains are discussed in greater detail below.

Translation of the human GRβ splice variant produces a 742 amino acid protein that differs from GRα only at the carboxy terminus (Fig. 1B). The two proteins are identical through amino acid 727, but then diverge with GRα having an additional 50 amino acids and GRβ an additional, nonhomologous 15 amino acids. Sequences in GRα that are important for ligand binding are partially disrupted in GRβ due to its unique carboxy-terminus. As a result, GRβ does not bind glucocorticoids and is currently classified as an orphan receptor [10, 14, 20]. GRβ-specific antibodies reveal expression of GRβ within a variety of human tissues [21], and immunoblots performed with antibodies that recognize the same epitope in both GRα and GRβ indicate that GRβ is expressed at lower levels than GRα [21]. However the relative levels of GRα and GRβ measured in tissues may not reflect the situation in individual cells, particularly since GRβ appears to be expressed in a cell-type specific pattern. GRβ is most abundant in certain epithelial cells, including those lining the terminal bronchiole of the lung, forming the outer layer of Hassall's corpuscle in the thymus, and lining the bile duct in the liver [21].

Function of GRα

GRα in the absence of ligand
In the absence of hormone, GRα exists as a large heteromeric complex consisting of the receptor polypeptide, two molecules of hsp90, and one molecule of the heat shock protein hsp56 [23, 24] (Fig. 2). The association of GRα with hsp90 maintains the receptor in a conformation that will not bind DNA, but will bind hormone with high affinity. The GRα-hsp90 interaction has been documented by many different laboratories using a variety of techniques. Identifying the amino acid residues within the receptor that contact hsp90 has proved more elusive. Analysis of mouse and rat GRα mutants with varying internal deletions and/or C-terminal truncations has shown that the amino-terminal half of the HBD is both essential and sufficient for hsp90 association [25, 26]. However, similar studies on human GRα have found that hsp90 interacts with multiple sites along the entire HBD [27] (Fig. 1B). hsp56 is a member of the immunophilin family of proteins that mediate the actions of the immunosuppressive drugs FK506 and rapamycin [28]. This protein associates with GRα *via* binding hsp90 and is thought to have an important role in protein folding [29].

One of the unique features of GRα that distinguishes it from other steroid hormone receptors is its subcellular distribution. GRα is generally thought to reside predominantly in the cytoplasm of cells in the absence of hormone and then translocate to the nucleus upon hormone binding (Fig. 2). Although results from many immunocytochemical studies support this view, a few studies have reported that GRα resides in the nucleus of cells independent of glu-

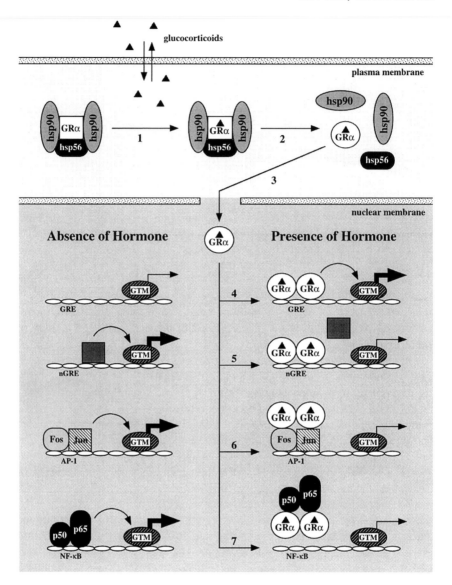

Figure 2. Schematic representation of the signal transduction pathway for glucocorticoids. Details for steps 1–7 are provided in the text. GTM, general transcription machinery.

cocorticoid treatment [30]. These divergent results are often attributed to differences in the fixation and/or permeabilization procedures utilized by the different laboratories. The use of non-selective antibodies that recognized both GRα and GRβ may also have contributed to the conflicting data since GRβ is found constitutively in the nucleus of cells [14, 21]. An antibody specific for

GRα has now been developed [31], and its use in immunocytochemical experiments has shown that GRα resides in the cytoplasm of cells in the absence of hormone and translocates to the nucleus in a hormone-dependent manner [31]. The controversy surrounding GRα's subcellular distribution may also indicate, however, that the compartmentalization of GRα differs in a cell-type specific manner or even within the same cell depending on its stage of development, degree of differentiation, and/or phase of the cell cycle.

Hormone binding, activation, and translocation of GRα
Glucocorticoids are lipophilic in nature and are thought to passively diffuse across the plasma membrane, although a few studies have suggested that an active uptake mechanism is involved [32, 33]. Once in the cell glucocorticoids bind with high affinity to GRα (Fig. 2, step 1). The HBD domain is comprised of the 250 C-terminal amino acids (Fig. 1B), and with few exceptions [34, 35], modification of this domain by deletion, truncation, or point mutation results in a reduction or complete loss of hormone binding [12, 36–38]. Some of the amino acids known to be important for ligand binding are quite remote from each other in the primary sequence suggesting that the HBD forms a hydrophobic pocket for the reception of ligand. In addition to binding glucocorticoids, the HBD functions as a repressor of the transcriptional activity of the receptor in the absence of ligand. Removal of the HBD results in a constitutively active receptor [39].

GRα undergoes a conformational change concomitant with hormone binding that results in the dissociation of the hsp90 and hsp56 molecules (Fig. 2, step 2). This poorly understood process is referred to as "receptor activation," conveying the idea that GRα can now bind DNA and activate transcription. The ligand-induced conformational change in the receptor has several functional consequences. One is that GRα becomes hyperphosphorylated. Multiple phosphorylation sites have been identified in the amino-terminal region of GRα, and hormone treatment increases phosphorylation at all of the sites [40, 41]. This post-translational modification appears to regulate the ability of GRα to activate gene transcription from certain promoters and also to regulate the stability of the GRα protein (see below). The change in conformation also results in rapid translocation of the receptor into the nucleus [30, 31] (Fig. 2, step 3). GRα contains two nuclear localization signals (NLS) designated NL1 and NL2 [42] (Fig. 1B). NL1 resides within a 27 amino acid segment found between the carboxy-terminus of the DBD and the amino-terminus of the HBD and is homologous to the SV40 T-antigen NLS. NL2 is located within the HBD. The association of hsp90 with GRα is thought to mask or inactivate these NLS in the absence of hormone [43, 44]. Dissociation of hsp90 from the receptor, induced by ligand binding or heat stress, results in the unmasking or activation of the NLS and translocation of GRα into the nucleus. Finally, the change in conformation accompanying hormone binding is also necessary for transcriptional activity. Heat and/or chemical stress as well as glucocorticoid antagonists such as RU 486 can drive the receptor into the nucleus where it can interact with DNA, but activation of gene expression does not occur in the absence of glucocorticoids [45, 46].

DNA binding

Activated GRα binds specific sequences of DNA called glucocorticoid responsive elements (GREs) that are located in the regulatory regions of target genes (Fig. 2, step 4). Analysis of many different glucocorticoid-responsive promoters has permitted the derivation of the following consensus GRE sequence: 5' GGTACAnnnTGTTCT 3' [47, 48]. This 15 base pair element is palindromic in nature, consisting of two half-sites separated by three base pairs. The three intervening bases can be any nucleotide, but the spacing of the three is invariant. Most natural GREs consist of one well-conserved half-site (usually the 3' site) and one that deviates considerably from the consensus. The amino acids that recognize and interact with the GRE are located in the GRα DBD (Fig. 1B). This domain is comprised of 66 amino acids and contains eight cysteines that are invariant throughout the nuclear receptor superfamily [48]. By tetrahedrally coordinating two zinc ions, these cysteine residues form two zinc fingers in the DBD. The zinc finger region is both necessary and sufficient for specific GRE binding. Mutagenesis has shown that the first finger is responsible for specific recognition of the GRE, and the second finger is involved in protein-protein interactions.

The palindromic nature of GREs suggested that GRα bound its response element as a dimer. Dimerization of GRα was subsequently demonstrated for both the intact receptor and a truncated receptor containing only the DBD [49–51]. Whether a preformed GRα dimer binds the GRE or whether dimerization occurs concurrent with DNA binding is still not clearly understood. Regions of the receptor involved in dimerization have been mapped to a five amino acid segment at the base of the second zinc finger known as the D-box and to a region in the HBD [52, 53] (Fig. 1B). The latter region has not been precisely mapped, but it is thought to reside near the carboxy-terminus. In support of this location, the major dimerization domain of the estrogen receptor (ER) has been shown to reside at the carboxy-terminal end of its HBD [54, 55]. The striking feature of this region in the ER is that it contains a heptad repeat of hydrophobic residues and this motif is highly conserved at the carboxy-terminal end of GRα. Dimerization is both necessary for high affinity binding of the receptor to the GRE and required for glucocorticoid-dependent induction of gene transcription [51, 56, 57].

Positive gene regulation

GRα when bound to the GRE stimulates transcription of target genes (Fig. 2, step 4). Although the DBD is required for gene activation, other regions of the molecule enhance the activation function. These regions are referred to as transactivation domains or transcriptional activation functions (TAF) and are defined as those portions of the receptor which, when combined with DNA binding activity, produce an increase in transcription initiation. Several transactivation domains have been identified for GRα (Fig. 1B) The major transactivation domain (tau 1 or TAF-1) is located in the amino-terminal region of the receptor [36, 58]. Tau 1 is 185 amino acids in length and can activate reporter genes when fused to the GRα DBD or to a heterologous DBD. Weaker transactivation domains have been described in the carboxy-terminal half of the receptor. Tau 2 is comprised of 30 amino acids located between the DBD and HBD [36, 58], and TAF-2 consists of 37 amino acid residues at the carboxy-terminus of GRα [59].

The receptor communicates, *via* its transactivation domains, with the basal transcription machinery to enhance transcription of the linked gene [60, 61]. Based on observations made for other members of the steroid hormone receptor subfamily, GRα may contact the general transcription machinery directly by interacting with the general transcription factor TFIIB [62]. More recent studies, however, indicate that the receptor contacts the general transcription machinery indirectly *via* protein-protein interactions with intermediary proteins termed coactivators [61, 63, 64]. Coactivators are bridging factors interposed between the receptor and the preinitiation complex that allow for efficient transcription of the target gene. Several coactivators have been identified that interact with GRα in a ligand-dependent manner and enhance transcription. These include SRC-1 (steroid receptor coactivator 1), GRIP1 (GR interacting protein 1), and the cAMP response element binding protein CBP [65–68]. Precisely how the direct or indirect interactions of the receptor with the basal transcription machinery result in an increase in transcription is unclear. For accurate initiation of transcription to occur, a number of general transcription factors as well as RNA polymerase II must assemble at the start site of transcription. Direct or indirect interactions between the transactivation domains of GRα and factors in this preinitiation complex might stimulate transcription by stabilizing the complex on the gene and/or by enhancing the recruitment of preformed complexes to the gene.

Eukaryotic DNA is organized in chromatin within the cell nucleus, and chromatin structure represses gene activity by denying transcription factors access to their cognate response elements. GRα has been shown to disrupt chromatin structure on several glucocorticoid responsive genes resulting in the binding of other transcription factors and the induction of gene expression [61]. The best-characterized example is the glucocorticoid-inducible mouse mammary tumor virus (MMTV) promoter, where binding of the receptor to the GRE initiates a rearrangement in the nucleosomes positioned around the response element [69]. This remodeling of chromatin structure allows the transcription factors NF1 (nuclear factor 1) and Oct-1 (octamer transcription factor 1) to bind the promoter and induce optimal levels of transcription. Thus, interaction of GRα with the structural components of chromatin appears to be another mechanism by which the receptor activates gene expression.

Negative gene regulation

GRα functions not only as an activator, but also as a repressor of gene expression. Negative regulation by glucocorticoids can be achieved by a direct interaction of GRα with a site on the DNA called a negative GRE (nGRE) [47, 70] (Fig. 2, step 5). The nGRE sequence is different from the classical, positive-acting GRE, but the nGREs so far described are too heterogeneous for a consensus sequence to be established. GRα-mediated repression of a number of genes including pro-opiomelanocortin, the alpha subunit of glycoprotein hormones, stromelysin, α-fetoprotein, prolactin, and osteocalcin involves receptor binding to an nGRE [71–75]. For each of these genes, an essential positive-acting transcription factor is thought to be either displaced from its cognate response element or prevented from binding to it by the interaction of the receptor with the neighboring nGRE. For example, GRα binds to a region overlapping the TATA box in the human osteocalcin gene suggesting that the receptor and TATA box binding factor (TFIID) compete for binding to the same site [75]. Many of these nGREs do not function as negative regulatory elements in response to glucocorticoids when placed in heterologous promoter systems indicating that additional cell-type specific factors and/or promoter sequences are involved.

GRα can also repress gene expression apart from DNA binding *via* protein-protein interactions with other transcription factors [64, 76–79] (Fig. 2, steps 6 and 7). For example, ligand-bound receptor can physically interact with the c-fos and c-jun components of AP-1 (activator protein-1) and inhibit the expression of the AP-1-responsive collagenase gene [80, 81]. This association does not prevent AP-1 from binding the collagenase promoter *in vivo* suggesting that GRα, when tethered to AP-1, interferes with the ability of AP-1 to interact with the general transcription machinery [82]. GRα also interferes with the transcriptional activity of NF-κB (nuclear factor-κB) *via* protein-protein interactions [83–86]. NF-κB is a heterodimer of 50 kDa (p50) and 65 kDa (p65 or rel A) subunits that functions as an activator of a broad class of immune system genes. Activated GRα down-regulates the transcription of many NF-κB-responsive genes by forming a complex with NF-κB and preventing it from binding its cognate response element. Repression of AP-1- and NF-κB-responsive genes requires the DBD of GRα but not GRE binding, suggesting it is this region of GRα that contacts the AP-1 and NF-κB molecules [84, 87]. Many genes encoding cytokines, cell adhesion molecules, and enzymes involved in the synthesis of inflammatory mediators are activated by NF-κB and AP-1. Protein-protein interactions between these transcription factors and GRα appear to be the major mechanism underlying the anti-inflammatory action of glucocorticoids.

Regulation of GRα expression and function

GRα is expressed in almost all tissues, but its level varies considerably among different tissues. Even within the same tissue, there is a pronounced variation in receptor expression [88]. Since many studies have shown that there is a direct correlation between the number of GRα molecules in a cell and the cell's sensitivity to glucocorticoids [89, 90], it becomes important to understand the factors that regulate GRα expression. Cellular responsiveness to glucocorticoids is also modulated by alterations in the potency with which GRα functions as a ligand-dependent transcription factor. At each step in the glucocorticoid signal transduction pathway factors might intervene that enhance or repress the ability of GRα to effectively regulate gene expression. The following section discusses many of the factors that have been shown to regulate either expression of GRα or the potency with which GRα functions as a ligand-dependent transcription factor.

Regulation of GRα expression

Homologous down-regulation
The best known and most intensively studied regulators of GRα expression are glucocorticoid hormones themselves. Glucocorticoid treatment of most cells and tissues results in a time- and dose-dependent reduction in the amount of GRα mRNA and protein by a process termed homologous down-regulation [91]. One exception are human T-cells which have been shown to upregulate their receptor mRNA and protein in response to glucocorticoids [92, 93]. The kinetics and magnitude of GRα down-regulation vary substantially among the systems investigated. A monophasic decrease in receptor levels to 20–50% of control values is observed in many cells. This reduction is either rapid (minimum levels reached after 2–12 h of glucocorticoid treatment) or more gradual (minimum levels reached after 48 h of glucocorticoid treatment). A cyclic or biphasic reduction in GRα levels is observed in other cells. Accompanying the decrease in receptor levels is a corresponding decrease in cellular sensitivity to glucocorticoids [94, 95]. Thus, homologous down-regulation is a negative feedback mechanism that protects cells from over-responding to the continued presence of ligand.

The tissue and cell-type specific differences in the kinetics and magnitude of down-regulation suggest that the mechanisms underlying this process are complex. Recent studies have demonstrated that ligand-bound GRα directly represses transcription of the GR gene [96, 97]. This reduction in transcription does not involve a glucocorticoid-inducible protein, occurs in the absence of the GR promoter, and requires DNA sequences within the coding region of the HBD (exons 5–9). These data suggest that the activated receptor binds an nGRE located in the coding region of the GR gene and inhibits transcription initiation. Similar "intragenic elements" mediate homologous down-regulation of the estrogen and androgen receptors [98–100]. Post-transcriptional and post-translational mechanisms also appear to be involved in GRα down-regulation [91]. The stability of the GRα mRNA transcripts and the stability of the GRα protein are both reduced following glucocorticoid treatment [97, 101–104]. To what extent these different mechanisms occur in the same cell is an important question that has not yet been answered. Tissue-specific and/or developmental stage-specific factors may favor one or another mechanism, allowing the cell to fine tune the kinetics and/or magnitude of the down-regulation process and modulate its responsiveness to glucocorticoids.

Phosphorylation

GRα is a phosphoprotein that contains multiple phosphorylation sites, and in the presence of hormone the basally phosphorylated receptor becomes hyperphosphorylated [40]. Recent work indicates that the phosphorylation status of the receptor has a profound effect on GRα expression [105]. In transfected cells, mutant mouse receptors lacking all eight phosphorylation sites have an extended half-life in the absence of hormone and are resistant to ligand-dependent destabilization. Wild-type GRα has a half-life of 18 h in the absence of hormone and a half-life of 9 h following glucocorticoid treatment. In contrast, dephosphorylated GRα has a half-life of 29 h in the absence of hormone and this value is not significantly altered by glucocorticoids. These results suggest that phosphorylation is important for receptor turnover, and that dephosphorylated GRα is either in a conformation that is resistant to degradation or missing the signal for degradation. The half-life of the endogenous GRα protein varies from 8 to 25 h in the absence of hormone depending on the cell-type [102–104]. Cell-type specific differences in the availability and/or activity of various kinases and phosphatases may account not only for this broad range in GRα stability, but also for differences in receptor levels and glucocorticoid responsiveness.

Activation of protein kinase A (PKA) also indirectly influences GRα expression. Activators of PKA elicit a 2.5-fold increase in receptor levels in rat hepatoma cells by prolonging the half-life of GRα mRNA transcripts from 4 h to 10 h [106]. This 2.5-fold induction of GRα expression also leads to a corresponding 2.5-fold enhancement of glucocorticoid responsiveness. The events leading from activation of PKA to stabilization of receptor message are not known, but would appear to involve phosphorylation of a protein specifically involved in GRα mRNA turnover. These events are also cell-type specific as activation of the PKA pathway in other cells does not alter GRα expression [107, 108].

Promoter activity

The GR promoter has features that place the receptor into a family of constitutively active housekeeping genes, and this is not surprising given the ubiquitous expression of the receptor. However, transcription of the GR gene may be subject to cell-type specific regulation since receptor levels vary considerably between and within tissues. Only recently have *cis* elements and transcription factors been identified that potentially play important roles in controlling the activity of the GR promoter. AP-1 sites are known to be important for constitutive, basal transcription of numerous genes, and a putative AP-1 site which differs by one nucleotide from the consensus AP-1 site is located in the GR promoter [109]. Although it is not yet clear whether AP-1 actually binds this site, studies have shown that when cells are treated with agents that stimulate AP-1 expression, an increase in receptor mRNA and protein is observed [109, 110]. Conversely, when cells are treated with agents that decrease AP-1 activity, receptor expression is reduced. Glucocorticoids were used in the latter case, suggesting that protein-protein interactions between the receptor and AP-1 lead to a reduction in AP-1 activity on the GR promoter and, consequently, a reduction in GR gene expression. It has also been demonstrated recently that the transcription factor AP-2 binds to and activates the GR promoter [111]. By modulating the activity of the GR promoter, variations in the cellular levels of AP-1 and/or AP-2 might account for the tissue-specific differences in GRα levels and glucocorticoid responsiveness.

Cell-type specific differences in receptor expression may also result from the use of different promoters rather than the modulation of one promoter. Expression of the mouse GR gene is controlled by three promoters (1A, 1B, and 1C) [15]. Promoters 1B and 1C are active to various degrees in many cell lines and tissues, but promoter 1A is active only in T lymphocytes and lymphatic tissues. Interestingly, it is in these tissues that glucocorticoids upregulate GRα expression and induce apoptosis [92, 93, 112]. The challenge of future research will be to determine whether the mouse GR promoters 1A and 1B have human counterparts and to identify the factors regulating the activity of each promoter. These promoters may play critical roles in regulating GRα levels, not only in specific cell-types, but also in specific stages of development.

Alterations in GR gene structure

Only a few structural changes in the GR gene have been described that directly influence receptor expression. Deletion of a splice site (5' donor site at end of exon 6) in one of the two GR alleles has been found in a patient with generalized glucocorticoid resistance [113]. This deletion apparently results in the expression of only one GR allele since RT-PCR analysis does not detect the mutant mRNA. As expected, the 50% decrease in GRα protein renders all tissues of this patient hyposensitive to glucocorticoids. A deletion in the GR gene abolishing receptor expression has also been observed in a human leukemia cell line that is resistant to glucocorticoids [114]. This deletion involved all or part of the GR gene and developed after treating cells initially sensitive to glucocorticoids with cytotoxic drugs often used in combination with glucocorticoids in the treatment of hematological cancers. The growth inhibitory and cytolytic actions of glucocorticoids on lymphoid cells has made them the drug of choice for treating various leukemias and lymphomas, however their effectiveness is frequently limited due to the development of glucocorticoid resistant tumors [3]. Whether these cytotoxic drugs induce GR gene deletions in leukemic cells *in vivo* and account for the acquired glucocorticoid resistance is presently unknown.

The only other known alteration in GR gene structure that directly alters receptor expression was artificially constructed. Genetically engineered mice deficient in GRα have been generated by targeted disruption of the GR gene [115]. Mice homozygous for the GR mutation are nonresponsive to glucocorticoids and exhibit profound physiological consequences. For example, these mice die several hours after birth from respiratory distress due to improper lung development. Mice heterozygous for the GR mutation, however, are able to survive. Negative feedback is also impaired in these knockout mice, resulting in elevated levels of ACTH and corticosterone. Furthermore, liver enzymes involved in gluconeogenesis are not induced and adrenal chromaffin cells are absent from the adrenal medulla despite the high levels of circulating glucocorticoids. These results confirm many of the physiological actions attributed to glucocorticoids. With advances being made in diagnosing glucocorticoid resistance, more naturally occurring mutations in the GR gene that alter its expression are likely to be forthcoming. Finding mutations in the GR promoter and/or 3'UTR will be especially profitable for understanding the importance these regions have in regulating GRα expression.

Regulation of GRα function

Protein-protein interactions with AP-1 and NF-κB

GRα inhibits the transcriptional activity of AP-1 and NF-κB *via* protein-protein interactions (see above). In a reciprocal manner, AP-1 and NF-κB antagonize the transcriptional activity of GRα. For example, overexpression of the c-jun and c-fos components of AP-1 leads to a marked reduction in GRα-induced gene expression from a variety of GRE-containing promoters [116, 117]. Similar results are obtained when endogenous AP-1 is activated in response to growth factors or phorbol esters. Direct interactions between GRα and AP-1 have been observed *in vitro* and are thought to account for the antagonism *in vivo*. A physical association between these two proteins, however, does not prevent the receptor from binding a GRE *in vivo*, suggesting that AP-1 interferes with the ability of GRα to communicate with the basal transcription machinery [118] (Fig. 2, step 6). The physiological significance of this interaction in regulating glucocorticoid responsiveness has been demonstrated in the developing chicken retina where changes in c-jun expression are inversely correlated with the transcriptional activity of GRα and glucocorticoid sensitivity [119]. Elevated levels and enhanced activity of AP-1 also appear to underlie the reduced responsiveness to glucocorticoids observed in some patients with glucocorticoid-resistant asthma [120].

The ability of NF-κB to inhibit the transcriptional activity of GRα is mediated by the p65 subunit of NF-κB [83–86]. The p50 subunit and other members of the NF-κB family appear to have no effect. NF-κB and activated GRα have been shown to physically associate *in vitro* and *in vivo*, but whether this interaction prevents the receptor from binding its response element on the target gene or results in the formation of a transcriptionally inactive complex on the DNA is not clear. A variety of agents including viral proteins, mitogens, and cytokines activate NF-κB, and several lines of evidence suggest that constitutive activation of NF-κB contributes to the malignant phenotype of tumor cells [121–123]. By antagonizing GRα, constitutively active NF-κB may make these neoplastic cells resistant to the growth inhibitory effects of glucocorticoids. Enhanced activity of NF-κB may also be responsible for the development of glucocorticoid resistance at the site of inflammation in cases of rheumatoid arthritis, asthma, and sepsis. Cytokines are elevated at sites of inflammation, and high concentrations of cytokines have been shown to antagonize the anti-inflammatory actions of glucocorticoids in a dose-dependent manner [2, 124].

Coactivators
Communication between ligand-bound GRα and the general transcription machinery involves both direct and indirect contacts. Indirect contacts are mediated by coactivators which serve as bridging factors between the receptor and the transcription initiation complex and are necessary for efficient transcription to occur [61, 63, 64]. Over the last several years a number of coactivators have been identified that interact with GRα in a ligand-dependent manner and potentiate its transcriptional activity on target genes. For example, GRIP1 physically associates with the TAF-2 domain at the carboxy-terminus of the activated receptor and stimulates GRα-mediated transcription when coexpressed with the receptor in yeast [66, 125]. The coactivator SRC-1, which is homologous to GRIP1, enhances the transcriptional activity of the receptor in mammalian cells [65]. Both these proteins exert similar effects on many other members of the steroid/thyroid/retinoic acid receptor superfamily.

Another recently identified coactivator of GRα is the cAMP response element binding protein, CBP. CBP interacts *in vivo* with the GRα HBD. When functional levels of CBP are reduced in cells, receptor-dependent activation of responsive genes is reduced in a dose-dependent manner [67, 68]. CBP is a general coactivator required for efficient transactivation by other nuclear receptors and by other transcription factors such as AP-1. This latter observation suggests that the mutual antagonism between GRα and AP-1 may be due to competition for a limiting pool of CBP [67]. Transcriptional activity of GRα in yeast is dependent on the yeast proteins SWI1, SWI2 and SWI3 [126]. The human homologue of these yeast proteins (hbrm) functions as a GRα coactivator and potentiates GRα-mediated induction of gene expression in mammalian cells [127]. The retinoblastoma protein (Rb) directly interacts with hbrm and further enhances the transcriptional activity of GRα [128]. Other proteins that function as coactivators for GRα include GRIP170 and hRPF1 (the human homologue of yeast RSP5) [129, 130]. In sum, the presence or absence of coactivators will profoundly influence cellular responsiveness to glucocorticoids by modulating the transcriptional activity of GRα. An important area of future research will be to identify the factors and processes that regulate the expression and/or activity of these coactivators.

Phosphorylation

GRα is a phosphoprotein that becomes hyperphosphorylated after binding hormone [41]. Eight phosphorylation sites have been identified on mouse GRα and all of them are located in the amino-terminal half of the receptor [41, 105]. Of these eight sites, six reside in the tau 1 transactivation domain and, within this domain, three of the phosphorylation sites are located in a highly acidic region necessary for maximum transcription initiation [131]. The concentration of phosphorylation sites in the major transactivation domain suggests that the phosphorylation status of the receptor will modulate its transcriptional potency. Early studies, however, reported that dephosphorylated receptors were only slightly less effective than the wild-type receptor in activating transcription [132, 133]. The glucocorticoid-responsive promoters utilized in these experiments were complex in the sense that they contained binding sites for other transcription factors such as NF1 and Oct1, and these ancillary proteins may have compensated for the impaired ability of the dephosphorylated receptor to activate transcription. More recent studies have in fact demonstrated that the ability of dephosphorylated GRα to activate a simple glucocorticoid-responsive promoter containing only two consensus GREs and a TATA box is severely compromised [105]. Thus, the phosphorylation status of the receptor does appear to influence its transcriptional activity but only on certain promoters. Additional support for the involvement of phosphorylation in the functioning of GRα comes from studies showing that ligand-induced hyperphosphorylation of GRα does not occur during the G2 phase of the cell cycle, a time when many cells are unresponsive to glucocorticoids [134].

GRβ

Alternative splicing of the human GR primary transcript produces a splice variant (GRβ) that differs from the wild-type receptor (GRα) only at the carboxy terminus (see above and Fig. 1, A and B). GRβ does not bind glucocorticoids or antiglucocorticoids and, by itself, does not activate or repress glucocorticoid-responsive genes [14, 36]. However, when co-expressed with GRα, GRβ inhibits the ability of the wild-type receptor to activate both complex and simple glucocorticoid-responsive promoters [14, 20, 135]. The dominant negative activity of GRβ has also been observed on some genes negatively regulated by glucocorticoids. GRβ can specifically bind GREs and can physically associate with GRα, suggesting that competition for GRE binding and/or the formation of transcriptionally impaired GRα-GRβ heterodimers underlies the observed antagonism [135]. More direct evidence that heterodimerization is critical for GRβ's dominant negative activity comes from the recent demonstration that removal of GRβ's unique carboxyl-terminal 15 amino acids, which comprise the distal half of a carboxyl-terminal dimerization domain (Fig. 1B), generates a truncated receptor that no longer represses the transcriptional activity of GRα [135]. Cells with elevated levels of GRβ (relative to GRα) have been found in patients with glucocorticoid resistance, suggesting that an imbalance in GRα and GRβ expression may underlie the pathogenesis of many clinical conditions associated with glucocorticoid insensitivity [136, 137].

Mutations in the GR HBD

Most natural mutations described for the GR gene that influence cellular sensitivity to glucocorticoids without changing receptor levels are located in exons encoding the HBD [7, 138]. These mutations alter the receptor's affinity for hormone. Since the ability of the receptor to function effectively as a ligand-dependent transcription factor correlates with its hormone binding affinity, changes in affinity lead to corresponding changes in glucocorticoid responsiveness. For example, the primary cause of generalized glucocorticoid resistance in man are point mutations in the HBD. Three individuals have been described with mutations at positions 559 (D559I), 641 (D641V), and 729 (V729I) that decrease the affinity of the receptor for hormone and result in a weaker activation of target genes [139, 140]. Analysis of the GR gene in human leukemia and multiple myeloma cell lines resistant to glucocorticoids has revealed a mutation in a splice site (the 3' acceptor site at the beginning of exon 8) within the HBD [141, 142]. Translation of this mutant mRNA produces a truncated protein missing approximately 100 amino acids at the carboxy-terminus. This protein would not be expected to bind glucocorticoids since removal of as few as 29 amino acids from the carboxy-terminus of GRα decreases receptor affinity for hormone by 10 000-fold [37]. This same mutation also appears to be responsible for the glucocorticoid resistance observed in ACTH-secreting small cell lung cancer cells [143]. While most modifications of the GRα HBD destroy ligand binding, a few point mutations have been generated by site directed mutagenesis that actually increase receptor affinity for hormone and lead to an enhanced activation of target genes [34, 35]. What role, if any, these mutations have in mediating glucocorticoid hypersensitivity *in vivo* is not known.

Association of hsp90 and hsp56 with GRα

The affinity of GRα for hormone is controlled not only by the composition of amino acids in the HBD, but also by the conformation of the GRα protein. Association of hsp90 with GRα maintains the receptor in a conformation that binds hormone with high affinity [144, 145]. Factors that prevent, disrupt, or alter the GRα-hsp90 heteromeric complex will cause consequent changes in hormone binding affinity and glucocorticoid responsiveness. The first evidence for this came from studies demonstrating that adequate levels of hsp90 are required for the biological activity of GRα in yeast [146]. A reduction in hsp90 expression resulted in hsp90-free receptors that were markedly deficient at activating target genes in the presence of hormone. Mutations in the hsp90 protein have also been generated that prevent proper assembly of the GRα-hsp90 heteromeric complex [147, 148]. These mutations impair receptor function by eliminating or reducing its capacity to bind hormone. Whether similar mutations exist *in vivo* and account for glucocorticoid resistance is unknown. Further support for the importance of hsp90 in regulating receptor activity comes from studies using geldanamycin, a putative tyrosine kinase inhibitor that binds hsp90 [149]. The interaction of geldanamycin with hsp90 alters the composition of the GRα-hsp90 heteromeric complex, resulting in a reduction in both GRα's affinity for hormone and its transcriptional activity.

The hsp56 component of the GRα-hsp90 heteromeric complex also has an important role in modulating glucocorticoid responsiveness. Treatment of cells with the immunosuppressive drug FK506 enhances glucocorticoid-dependent gene expression [150, 151]. This potentiation has been attributed to an increase in hormone binding affinity mediated by FK506's interaction with hsp56.

Vitamin B6

Vitamin B_6 is a water soluble vitamin that plays critical roles in intermediary metabolism and is essential for normal growth and development. This nutrient alters the structure and DNA binding properties of GRα *in vitro* and modulates GRα activity *in vivo* [152]. Variations in the intracellular concentration of pyridoxal 5'-phosphate, the biologically active form of vitamin B_6, have pronounced effects on the ability of ligand-bound receptor to activate the glucocorticoid-responsive MMTV promoter [153]. Elevation of intracellular levels of pyridoxal 5'-phosphate results in a two- to three-fold increase in GRα-mediated induction of gene expression. Conversely, vitamin B_6 deficiency reduces the transcriptional activity of the receptor by 50%. This modulatory action of vitamin B_6 also occurs on other members of the steroid hormone receptor subfamily, but is promoter specific [154]. Glucocorticoid-induced gene expression from a simple promoter containing only two consensus GREs and TATA box is not affected by alterations in pyridoxal 5'-phosphate. However, inclusion of an NF1 binding site in the simple promoter restores the effects of vitamin on receptor-induced gene expression [155]. Therefore, it appears that vitamin B_6 influences a functional or cooperative interaction between GRα and the transcription factor NF1 that ultimately leads to changes in transcription initiation. Intracellular pyridoxal 5'-phosphate concentration varies greatly in the tissues and cells in which it has been measured, and variations in the concentration of this nutrient may serve as a mechanism through which local response to hormone is regulated in a cell-type specific manner.

Calreticulin

Calreticulin is a ubiquitously expressed calcium-binding protein that is found primarily in the endoplasmic reticulum, but also in the cytoplasm and nucleus. This protein is multifunctional and appears to be involved in many physiological processes. Calreticulin binds *in vitro* to a conserved amino acid sequence located between the two zinc fingers of the GRα DBD and prevents this receptor from binding its response element [156]. When overexpressed in cells containing endogenous GRα, calreticulin blocks the ability of GRα to activate both transfected and endogenous glucocorticoid-responsive genes. Calreticulin has similar effects on other members of the nuclear receptor superfamily [157, 158]. Whether a direct interaction between calreticulin and the GRα DBD occurs *in vivo* and accounts for the inhibition is controversial [159]. Differential expression of calreticulin provides yet another level at which GRα-mediated gene transcription can be regulated.

Conclusion

A variety of factors have now been identified that regulate cellular sensitivity to glucocorticoids by altering either GRα expression and/or the potency with which GRα functions as a ligand-dependent transcription factor. Elucidating the precise mechanisms by which these factors regulate the receptor as well as determining the role these factors play in physiological and pathophysiological changes in glucocorticoid responsiveness are challenges for future research. Insight into these issues will ultimately lead to the development of pharmacological agents that can modulate receptor levels and/or activity in a tissue-specific fashion. Such technology will greatly improve the prognosis of patients with, for example, acute leukemia, malignant lymphoma, asthma, and rheumatoid arthritis who develop resistance to glucocorticoid therapy.

References

1 Evans RM (1988) The steroid and thyroid hormone receptor superfamily. *Science* 240: 889–895
2 Lamberts SWJ, Huizenga ATM, de Lange P, de Jong FH, Koper JW (1996) Clinical aspects of glucocorticoid sensitivity. *Steroids* 61: 157–160
3 Sluyser M (1994) Hormone resistance in cancer: the role of abnormal steroid receptors. *Crit Rev Oncogen* 5: 539–554
4 Gorovits R, Ben-Dror I, Fox LE, Westphal HM, Vardimon L (1994) Developmental changes in the expression and compartmentalization of the glucocorticoid receptor in embryonic retina. *Proc Natl Acad Sci USA* 91: 4786–4790
5 Hsu S, DeFranco DB (1995) Selectivity of cell cycle regulation of glucocorticoid receptor function. *J Biol Chem* 270: 3359–3364
6 Bamberger CM, Schulte HM, Chrousos GP (1996) Molecular determinants of glucocorticoid receptor function and tissue sensitivity to glucocorticoids. *Endocrine Rev* 17: 245–261
7 Bronnegard M, Stierna P, Marcus C (1996) Glucocorticoid resistant syndromes – molecular basis and clinical presentations. *J Neuroendocrinol* 8: 405–415
8 Ballard PL, Baxter JD, Higgins SJ, Rousseau GG, Tomkins GM (1974) General presence of glucocorticoid receptors in mammalian cells. *Endocrinology* 94: 998–1002
9 Mangelsdorf DJ, Thummel C, Beato M, Herrlich P, Schutz G, Umesono K, Blumberg B, Kastner P, Mark M, Chambon P, Evans RM (1995) The nuclear receptor superfamily: the second decade. *Cell* 83: 835–839
10 Hollenberg SM, Weinberger C, Ong ES, Cerelli G, Oro A, Lebo R, Thompson EB, Rosenfeld MG, Evans RM (1985) Primary structure and expression of a functional human glucocorticoid receptor cDNA. *Nature* 318: 635–641

11 Miesfeld R, Rusconi S, Godowski PJ, Maler BA, Okret S, Wikstrom A-C, Gustafsson J-A, Yamamoto KR (1986) Genetic complementation of a glucocorticoid receptor deficiency by expression of cloned receptor cDNA. *Cell* 46: 389–399

12 Danielsen M, Northrop JP, Ringold GM (1986) The mouse glucocorticoid receptor: mapping of functional domains by cloning, sequencing and expression of wild-type and mutant receptor proteins. *EMBO J* 5: 2513–2522

13 Encio IJ, Detera-Wadleigh SD (1991) The genomic structure of the human glucocorticoid receptor. *J Biol Chem* 266: 7182–7188

14 Oakley RH, Sar M, Cidlowski JA (1996) The human glucocorticoid receptor beta isoform: expression, biochemical properties, and putative function. *J Biol Chem* 271: 9550–9559

15 Strahle U, Schmidt A, Kelsey G, Stewart AF, Cole TJ, Schmid W, Schutz G (1992) At least three promoters direct expression of the mouse glucocorticoid receptor gene. *Proc Natl Acad Sci USA* 89: 6731–6735

16 Zong J, Ashraf J, Thompson EB (1990) The promoter and first, untranslated exon of the human glucocorticoid receptor gene are GC rich but lack consensus glucocorticoid receptor element sites. *Mol Cell Biol* 10: 5580–5585

17 Govindan MV, Pothier F, LeClerc S, Palaniswami R, Xie B (1991) Human glucocorticoid receptor gene promoter – homolgous down regulation. *J Steroid Biochem Mol Biol* 40: 317–323

18 Swick A, Blake MC, Kahn JW, Azizkhan JC (1989) Functional analysis of GC element binding and transcription in the hamster dihydrofolate reductase gene promoter. *Nucl Acid Res* 17: 9291–9304

19 Gearing KL, Cairns W, Okret S, Gustafsson J-A (1993) Heterogeneity in the 5' untranslated region of the rat glucocorticoid receptor mRNA. *J Steroid Biochem Mol Biol* 46: 635–639

20 Bamberger CM, Bamberger A-M, de Castro M, Chrousos GP (1995) Glucocorticoid receptor β, a potential endogenous inhibitor of glucocorticoid action in humans. *J Clin Invest* 95: 2435–2441

21 Oakley RH, Webster JC, Sar M, Parker CR, Cidlowski JA (1997) Expression and subcellular distribution of the beta isoform of the human glucocorticoid receptor. *Endocrinology* 138: 5028–5038

22 Otto C, Reichardt HM, Schutz G (1997) Absence of glucocorticoid receptor beta in mice. *J Biol Chem* 272: 26665–26668

23 Pratt WB (1993) The role of the heat shock proteins in regulating the function, folding, and trafficking of the glucocorticoid receptor. *J Biol Chem* 268: 21455–21458

24 Smith DF, Toft DO (1993) Steroid receptors and their associated proteins. *Mol Endocrinol* 7: 4–11

25 Howard KJ, Holley SJ, Yamamoto KR, Distelhorst CW (1990) Mapping the hsp90 binding region of the glucocorticoid receptor. *J Biol Chem* 265: 11928–11935

26 Dalman FC, Scherrer LC, Taylor LP, Akil H, Pratt WB (1991) Localization of the 90-kDa heat shock protein-binding site within the hormone-binding domain of the glucocorticoid receptor by peptide competition. *J Biol Chem* 266: 3482–3490

27 Cadepond F, Schweizer-Groyer G, Segard-Maurel I, Jibard N, Hollenberg SM, Giguere V, Evans RM, Baulieu E-E (1991) Heat shock protein 90 as a critical factor in maintaining glucocorticosteroid receptor in a nonfunctional state. *J Biol Chem* 266: 5834–5841

28 Tai PKK, Albers MW, Chang H, Faber LE, Schreiber SL (1992) Association of a 59-kilodalton immunophilin and the glucocorticoid receptor complex. *Science* 256: 1315–1318

29 Renoir JM, Radanyi C, Faber LE, Baulieu EE (1990) The non DNA-binding heterooligomeric form of mammalian steroid hormone receptors contains a hsp90-bound 59-kilodalton protein. *J Biol Chem* 265: 10740–10745

30 Webster JC, Jewell CM, Sar M, Cidlowski JA (1994) The glucocorticoid receptor: maybe not all steroid receptors are nuclear. *Endocrine* 2: 967–969

31 Oakley RH, Webster JC, Jewell CM, Sar M, Cidlowski JA (1999) Immunocytochemical analysis of the glucocorticoid receptor alpha isoform (GRα) using a GRα-specific antibody. *Steroids* 64: 742–751

32 Harrison RW, Fairfield S, Orth DN (1974) Evidence for glucocorticoid transport through the target cell membrane. *Biochem Biophys Res Commun* 61: 1262–1267

33 Rao ML, Rao GS, Eckel J, Breuer H (1977) Factors involved in the uptake of corticosterone by rat liver cells. *Biochim Biophys Acta* 500: 322–332

34 Chakraborti PK, Garabedian MJ, Yamamoto KR, Simons SSJr, (1991) Creation of "super" glucocorticoid receptors by point mutations in the steroid binding domain. *J Biol Chem* 266: 22075–22078

35 Warriar N, Yu C, Govindan MV (1994) Hormone binding domain of the human glucocorticoid receptor. *J Biol Chem* 269: 29010–29015
36 Giguere V, Hollenberg SM, Rosenfeld MG, Evans RM (1986) Functional domains of the human glucocorticoid receptor. *Cell* 46: 645–652
37 Rusconi S, Yamamoto KR (1987) Functional dissection of the hormone and DNA binding activities of the glucocorticoid receptor. *EMBO J* 6: 1309–1315
38 Hurley DM, Accili D, Stratikis CA, Karl M, Vamvakopoulos N, Rorer E, Constantine K, Taylor SI, Chrousos GP (1991) Point mutation causing a single amino acid substitution in the hormone binding domain of the glucocorticoid receptor in familial glucocorticoid resistance. *J Clin Invest* 87: 680–686
39 Godowski PJ, Rusconi S, Miesfeld R, Yamamoto KR (1987) Glucocorticoid receptor mutants that are constitutive activators of transcriptional enhancement. *Nature* 325: 365–368
40 Orti E, Mendel DB, Smith LI, Munck A (1989) Agonist-dependent phosphorylation and nuclear dephosphorylation of glucocorticoid receptors in intact cells. *J Biol Chem* 264: 9728–9731
41 Bodwell JE, Orti E, Coull JM, Pappin DJC, Smith LI, Swift F (1991) Identification of phosphorylated sites in the mouse glucocorticoid receptor. *J Biol Chem* 266: 7549–7555
42 Picard D, Yamamoto KR (1987) Two signals mediate hormone-dependent nuclear localization of the glucocorticoid receptor. *EMBO J* 6: 3333–3340
43 Picard D, Salser SJ, Yamamoto KR (1988) A movable and regulable inactivation function within the steroid binding domain of the glucocorticoid receptor. *Cell* 54: 1073–1080
44 Scherrer LC, Picard D, Massa E, Harmon JM, Simons SS, Yamamoto KR, Pratt WB (1993) Evidence that the hormone binding domain of steroid receptors confers hormonal control on chimeric proteins by determining their hormone-regulated binding to heat-shock protein 90. *Biochemistry* 32: 5381–5386
45 Sanchez ER, Hu JL, Zhong SJ, Shen P, Greene MJ, Housley PR (1994) Potentiation of glucocorticoid receptor-mediated gene expression by heat and chemical shock. *Mol Endocrinol* 8: 408–421
46 Mao J, Regelson W, Kalimi M (1992) Molecular mechanism of RU 486 action: a review. *Mol Cell Biochem* 109: 1–8
47 Beato M (1989) Gene regulation by steroid hormones. *Cell* 56: 335–344
48 Freedman LP (1992) Anatomy of the steroid receptor zinc finger region. *Endocrine Rev* 13: 129–145
49 Wrange O, Eriksson P, Perlmann T (1989) The purified activated glucocorticoid receptor is a homodimer. *J Biol Chem* 264: 5253–5259
50 Dahlman-Wright K, Siltala-Roos H, Carlstedt-Duke J, Gustafsson J-A (1990) Protein-protein interactions facilitate DNA binding by the glucocorticoid receptor DNA-binding domain. *J Biol Chem* 265: 14030–14035
51 Cairns W, Cairns C, Pongratz I, Poellinger L, Okret S (1991) Assembly of a glucocorticoid receptor complex prior to DNA binding enhances its specific interaction with a glucocorticoid response element. *J Biol Chem* 266: 11221–11226
52 Dahlman-Wright K, Wright A, Gustafsson J-A, Carlstedt-Duke J (1991) Interaction of the glucocorticoid receptor DNA-binding domain with DNA as a dimer is mediated by a short segment of five amino acids. *J Biol Chem* 266: 3107–3112
53 Dahlman-Wright K, Wright APH, Gustafsson J-A (1992) Determinants of high affinity DNA binding by the glucocorticoid receptor: evaluation of receptor domains outside the DNA-binding domain. *Biochemistry* 31: 9040–9044
54 Kumar V, Chambon P (1988) The estrogen receptor binds tightly to its responsive element as a ligand-induced homodimer. *Cell* 55: 145–156
55 Farwell SE, Lees JA, White R, Parker MG (1990) Characterization and localization of steroid binding and dimerization activities in the mouse estrogen receptor. *Cell* 60: 953–962
56 Perlmann T, Eriksson P, Wrange O (1990) Quantitative analysis of the glucocorticoid receptor-DNA interaction at the mouse mammary tumor virus glucocorticoid response element. *J Biol Chem* 265: 17222–17229
57 Drouin J, Sun YL, Tremblay S, Lavender P, Schmidt TJ, de Lean A, Nemer M (1992) Homodimer formation is rate-limiting for high affinity DNA binding by glucocorticoid receptor. *Mol Endocrinol* 6: 1299–1309
58 Hollenberg SM, Evans RM (1988) Multiple and cooperative transactivation domains of the human glucocorticoid receptor. *Cell* 55: 899–906
59 Danielian PS, White R, Lees JA, Parker MG (1992) Identification of a conserved region required

for hormone dependent transcriptional activation by steroid hormone receptors. *EMBO J* 11: 1025–1033

60 Truss M, Beato M (1993) Steroid hormone receptors: interaction with deoxyribonucleic acid and transcription factors. *Endocrine Rev* 14: 459–479

61 Beato M, Sanchez-Pacheco A (1996) Interaction of steroid hormone receptors with the transcription initiation complex. *Endocrine Rev* 17: 587–609

62 Ing NH, Beekman JM, Tsai SY, Tsai MJ, O'Malley BW (1992) Members of the steroid hormone receptor superfamily interact with TFIIB (S300-II). *J Biol Chem* 267: 17617–17623

63 Horwitz KB, Jackson TA, Bain DL, Richer JK, Takimoto GS, Tung L (1996) Nuclear receptor coactivators and corepressors. *Mol Endocrinol* 10: 1167–1177

64 McEwan IJ, Wright APH, Gustafsson J-A (1997) Mechanism of gene expression by the glucocorticoid receptor: role for protein-protein interactions. *BioEssays* 19: 153–160

65 Onate SA, Tsai SY, Tsai M-J, O'Malley BW (1995) Sequence and characterization of a coactivator for the steroid hormone receptor superfamily. *Science* 270: 1354–1357

66 Hong H, Kohli K, Trivedi A, Johnson DL, Stallcup MR (1996) GRIP1, a novel mouse protein that serves as a transcriptional coactivator in yeast for the hormone binding domains of steroid receptors. *Proc Natl Acad Sci USA* 93: 4948–4952

67 Kamei Y, Xu L, Heinzel T, Torchia J, Kurokawa R, Gloss B, Lin SC, Heyman RA, Rose DW, Glass CK, Rosenfeld MG (1996) A CBP integrator complex mediates transcriptional activation and AP-1 inhibition by nuclear receptors. *Cell* 85: 403–414

68 Chakravarti D, LaMorte VJ, Nelson MC, Nakajima T, Schulman IG, Juguilon H, Montminy M, Evans RM (1996) Role of CBP/P300 in nuclear receptor signalling. *Nature* 383: 99–103

69 Truss M, Bartsch J, Schelbert A, Hache RJG, Beato M (1995) Hormone induces binding of receptors and transcription factors to a rearranged nucleosome on the MMTV promoter *in vivo*. *EMBO J* 14: 1737–1751

70 Cairns C, Cairns W, Okret S (1993) Inhibition of gene expression by steroid hormone receptors *via* a negative glucocorticoid response element: evidence for the involvement of DNA-binding and agonistic effects of the antiglucocorticoid/antiprogestin RU 486. *DNA Cell Biol* 12: 695–702

71 Drouin J, Trifiro MA, Plante RK, Nemer M, Eriksson P, Wrange O (1989) Glucocorticoid receptor binding to a specific DNA sequence is required for hormone-dependent repression of proopiomelanocortin gene transcription. *Mol Cell Biol* 9: 5305–5314

72 Akerblom IW, Slater EP, Beato M, Baxter JD, Mellon PL (1988) Negative regulation by glucocorticoids through interference with a cAMP responsive enhancer. *Science* 241: 350–353

73 Guertin M, LaRue H, Bernier D, Wrange O, Chevrette M, Gingras M-C, Belanger L (1988) Enhancer and promoter elements directing activation and glucocorticoid repression of the α1-fetoprotein gene in hepatocytes. *Mol Cell Biol* 8: 1398–1407

74 Sakai DD, Helms S, Carlstedt-Duke J, Gustafsson JA, Rottman FM, Yamamoto KR (1988) Hormone-mediated repression of transcription: a negative glucocorticoid response element from the bovine prolactin gene. *Gene Develop* 2: 1144–1154

75 Stromstedt P-E, Poellinger L, Gustafsson J-A, Carlstedt-Duke J (1991) The glucocorticoid receptor binds to a sequence overlapping the TATA box of the human osteocalcin promoter: a potential mechanism of negative regulation. *Mol Cell Biol* 11: 3379–3383

76 Cato ACB, Wade E (1996) Molecular mechanisms of anti-inflammatory action of glucocorticoids. *BioEssays* 18: 371–378

77 Barnes PJ, Karin M (1997) Nuclear factor-κB-a pivotal transcription factor in chronic inflammatory diseases. *N Engl J Med* 336: 1066–1071

78 McKay LI, Cidlowski JA (1999) Molecular control of immune/inflammatory responses: interactions between NF-κB and steroid receptor signaling pathways. *Endocrine Rev* 20: 435–459

79 Beato M, Herrlich P, Schutz G (1995) Steroid hormone receptors: many actors in search of a plot. *Cell* 83: 851–857

80 Jonat C, Rahmsdorf HJ, Park KK, Cato AC, Gebel S, Ponta H, Herrlich P (1990) Antitumor promotion and anti-inflammation: down-modulation of AP-1 (fos/jun) activity by glucocorticoid hormone. *Cell* 62: 1189–1204

81 Schule R, Rangarajan P, Kliewer S, Ransone LJ, Bolado J, Yang N, Verma IM, Evans RM (1990) Functional antagonism between oncoprotein c-Jun and the glucocorticoid receptor. *Cell* 62: 1217–1226

82 Konig H, Ponta H, Rahmsdorf HJ, Herrlich P (1992) Interference between pathway specific transcription factors: glucocorticoids antagonize phorbol ester-induced AP-1 activity without altering

AP-1 site occupation *in vivo. EMBO J* 11: 2241–2246

83 Ray A, Prefontaine KE (1994) Physical association and functional antagonism between the p65 subunit of transcription factor NF-kappa B and the glucocorticoid receptor. *Proc Natl Acad Sci USA* 91: 752–756

84 Caldenhoven E, Liden J, Wissink S, Van de Stolpe A, Raaijmakers J, Koenderman L, Okret S, Gustafsson J-A, Van der Saag PT (1995) Negative cross-talk between RelA and the glucocorticoid receptor: a possible mechanism of the antiinflammatory action of glucocorticoids. *Mol Endocrinol* 9: 401–412

85 Scheinman RI, Gualberto A, Jewell CM, Cidlowski JA, Baldwin AS (1995) Characterization of mechanisms involved in transrepression of NF-κB by activated glucocorticoid receptors. *Mol Cell Biol* 15: 943–953

86 McKay LI, Cidlowski JA (1999) Cross-talk between nuclear factor-κB and the steroid hormone receptors: mechanisms of mutual antagonism. *Mol Endocrinol* 12: 45–56

87 Heck S, Kullmann M, Gast A, Ponta H, Rahmsdorf HJ, Herrlich P, Cato ACB (1994) A distinct modulating domain in glucocorticoid receptor monomers in repression of activity of the transcription factor AP-1. *EMBO J* 13: 4087–4095

88 Herman JP, Patel PD, Akil H, Watson SJ (1989) Localization and regulation of glucocorticoid and mineralocorticoid receptor messenger RNAs in the hippocampal formation of the rat. *Mol Endocrinol* 3: 1886–1894

89 Gehring U, Mugele K, Ulrich J (1984) Cellular receptor levels and glucocorticoid responsiveness of lymphoma cells. *Mol Cell Endocrinol* 36: 107–112

90 Vanderbilt JN, Miesfeld R, Maler BA, Yamamoto KR (1987) Intracellular receptor concentration limits glucocorticoid-dependent enhancer activity. *Mol Endocrinol* 1: 68–76

91 Oakley RH, Cidlowski JA (1993) Homologous down regulation of the glucocorticoid receptor: the molecular machinery. *Crit Rev Eukaryotic. Gene Expr* 3: 63–88

92 Eisen LP, Elsasser MS, Harmon JM (1988) Positive regulation of the glucocorticoid receptor in human T-cells sensitive to the cytolytic effects of glucocorticoids. *J Biol Chem* 263: 12044–12048

93 Denton RR, Eisen LP, Elsasser MS, Harmon JM (1993) Differential autoregulation of glucocorticoid receptor expression in human T- and B-cell lines. *Endocrinology* 133: 248–256

94 Yi Li Y, Jin-Xing T, Ren-Bao X (1989) Down-regulation of glucocorticoid receptor and its relationship to the induction of rat liver tyrosine aminotransferase. *J Steroid Biochem* 32: 99–104

95 Bellingham DL, Sar M, Cidlowski JA (1992) Ligand-dependent down regulation of stably transfected human glucocorticoid receptors is associated with the loss of functional glucocorticoid responsiveness. *Mol Endocrinol* 6: 2090–2102

96 Burnstein KL, Jewell CM, Cidlowski JA (1990) Human glucocorticoid receptor cDNA contains sequences sufficient for receptor down-regulation. *J Biol Chem* 265: 7284–7291

97 Burnstein KL, Jewell CM, Sar M, Cidlowski JA (1994) Intragenic sequences of the human glucocorticoid receptor complementary DNA mediate hormone-inducible receptor messenger RNA down-regulation through multiple mechanisms. *Mol Endocrinol* 8: 1764–1773

98 Kaneko KJ, Furlow JD, Gorski J (1993) Involvement of the coding sequence for the estrogen receptor gene in autologous ligand-dependent down-regulation. *Mol Endocrinol* 7: 879–888

99 Burnstein KL, Maiorino CA, Dai JL, Cameron DJ (1995) Androgen and glucocorticoid regulation of androgen receptor cDNA expression. *Mol Cell Endocrinol* 115: 177–186

100 Dai JL, Burnstein KL (1996) Two androgen response elements in the androgen receptor coding region are required for cell-specific up-regulation of receptor messenger RNA. *Mol Endocrinol* 10: 1582–1594

101 Vedeckis WV, Ali M, Allen HR (1989) Regulation of glucocorticoid receptor protein and mRNA levels. *Cancer Res (Suppl)* 49: 2295–2301

102 McIntyre WR, Samuels HH (1985) Triamcinolone acetonide regulates glucocorticoid receptor levels by decreasing the half-life of the activated nuclear receptor form. *J Biol Chem* 260: 418–427

103 Dong Y, Poellinger L, Gustafsson J-A, Okret S (1988) Regulation of glucocorticoid receptor expression: evidence for transcriptional and posttranslational mechanisms. *Mol Endocrinol* 2: 1256–1264

104 Hoeck W, Rusconi S, Groner B (1989) Down-regulation and phosphorylation of glucocorticoid receptor in cultured cells. *J Biol Chem* 264: 14396–14402

105 Webster JC, Jewell CM, Bodwell JE, Munck A, Sar M, Cidlowski JA (1997) Mouse glucocorti-

coid receptor phosphorylation status influences multiple functions of the receptor protein. *J Biol Chem* 272: 9287–9293

106 Dong Y, Aronsson M, Gustafsson J-A, Okret S (1989) The mechanism of cAMP-induced glucocorticoid receptor expression. *J Biol Chem* 264: 13679–13683

107 Rangarajan PN, Umesono K, Evans RM (1992) Modulation of glucocorticoid receptor function by protein kinas A. *Mol Endocrinol* 6: 1451–1457

108 Moyer ML, Borror KC, Bona BJ, DeFranco DB, Nordeen SK (1993) Modulation of cell signaling pathways can enhance or impair glucocorticoid-induced gene expression without altering the sate of receptor phosphorylation. *J Biol Chem* 268: 22933–22940

109 Vig E, Barrett TJ, Vedeckis WV (1994) Coordinate regulation of glucocorticoid receptor and c-jun mRNA levels: evidence for cross-talk between two signaling pathways at the transcriptional level. *Mol Endocrinol* 8: 1336–1346

110 Barrett TJ, Vig E, Vedeckis WV (1996) Coordinate regulation of glucocorticoid receptor and c-jun gene expression is cell type-specific and exhibits differential hormonal sensitivity for down- and up-regulation. *Biochemistry* 35: 9746–9753

111 Nobukuni Y, Smith CL, Hager GL, Detera-Wadleigh SD (1995) Characterization of the human glucocorticoid receptor promoter. *Biochemistry* 34: 8207–8214

112 Compton MM, Cidlowski JA (1987) Identification of a glucocorticoid induced nuclease in thymocytes: a potential "lysis gene" product. *J Biol Chem* 262: 8288–8292

113 Karl M, Lamberts SW, Detera-Wadleigh SD, Encio IJ, Stratakis CA, Hurley DM, Accili D, Chrousos GP (1993) Familial glucocorticoid resistance caused by a splice site deletion in the human glucocorticoid receptor gene. *J Clin Endocrinol Metab* 76: 683–689

114 Palmer LA, Hukku B, Harmon JM (1992) Human glucocorticoid receptor gene deletion following exposure to cancer chemotherapeutic drugs and chemical mutagens. *Cancer Res* 52: 6612–6618

115 Cole TJ, Blendy JA, Monaghan AP, Krieglstein K, Schmid W, Aguzzi A, Fantuzzi G, Hummler E, Unsicker K, Schutz G (1995) Targeted disruption of the glucocorticoid receptor blocks adrenergic chromaffin cell development and severely retards lung maturation. *Gene Develop* 9: 1608–1621

116 Pfahl M (1993) Nuclear receptor/AP-1 interaction. *Endocrine Rev* 14: 651–658

117 Herrlich P, Ponta H (1994) Mutual cross-modulation of steroid/retinoic acid receptor and AP-1 transcription factor activities. *Trends Endocrinol Metab* 5: 341–346

118 Reik A, Stewart AF, Schutz G (1994) Cross-talk modulation of signal transduction pathways: two mechanisms are involved in the control of tyrosine aminotransferase gene expression by phorbol esters. *Mol Endocrinol* 8: 490–497

119 Berko-Flint Y, Levkowitz G, Vardimon L (1994) Involvement of c-Jun in the control of glucocorticoid receptor transcription activity during development of chicken retinal tissue. *EMBO J* 13: 646–654

120 Adcock IM, Lane SJ, Brown CR, Lee TH, Barnes PJ (1995) Abnormal glucocorticoid receptor-activator protein 1 interaction in steroid-resistant asthma. *J Exp Med* 182: 1951–1958

121 Narayanan R, Klement JF, Ruben SM, Higgins KA, Rosen CA (1992) Identification of a naturally occurring transforming variant of the p65 subunit of NF-kappa B. *Science* 256: 367–370

122 Higgins KA, Perez JR, Coleman TA, Dorshkind K, McComas WA, Sarmiento UM, Rosen CA, Narayanan R (1993) Antisense inhibition of the p65 subunit of NF-kappa B blocks tumorigenicity and causes tumor regression. *Proc Natl Acad Sci USA* 90: 9901–9905

123 Beauparlant P, Kwan I, Bitar R, Chou P, Koromilas AE, Sonenberg N, Hiscott J (1994) Disruption of I kappa B alpha regulation by antisense RNA expression leads to malignant transformation. *Oncogene* 9: 3189–3197

124 Molijn GJ, Spek JJ, van Uffelen JCJ, de Jong FH, Brinkmann AO, Bruining HA, Lamberts SWJ (1995) Differential adaptation of glucocorticoid sensitivity of peripheral bood mononuclear leucocytes in patients with sepsis or septic shock. *J Clin Endocrinol Metab* 80: 1799–1803

125 Hong H, Kohli K, Garabedian MJ, Stallcup MR (1997) GRIP1, a transcriptional coactivator for the AF-2 transactivation domain of steroid, thyroid, retinoid, and vitamin D receptors. *Mol Cell Biol* 17: 2735–2744

126 Yoshinaga SK, Peterson CL, Herskowitz I, Yamamoto KR (1992) Roles of SWI1, SWI2, and SWI3 proteins for transcriptional enhancement by steroid receptors. *Science* 258: 1598–1604

127 Muchardt C, Yaniv M (1993) A human homologue of Saccharomyces cerevisiae SNF2/SWI2 and Drososphila brm genes potentiates transcriptional activation by the glucocorticoid receptor.

EMBO J 12: 4279–4290

128 Singh P, Coe J, Hong W (1995) A role for retinoblastoma protein in potentiating transcriptional activation by the glucocorticoid receptor. *Nature* 374: 562–565

129 Eggert M, Mows CC, Tripier D, Arnold R, Michel J, Nickel J, Schmidt S, Beato M, Renkawitz R (1995) A fraction enriched in a novel glucocorticoid receptor-interacting protein stimulates receptor-dependent transcription *in vitro*. *J Biol Chem* 270: 30755–30759

130 Imhof MO, McDonnell DP (1996) Yeast RSP5 and its human homolog hRPF1 potentiate hormone-dependent activation of transcription by human progesterone and glucocorticoid receptors. *Mol Cell Biol* 16: 2594–2605

131 Danielsen M, Northrop JP, Jonklaas J, Ringold GM (1987) Domains of the glucocorticoid receptor involved in specific and nonspecific deoxyribonucleic acid binding, hormone activation, and transcriptional enhancement. *Mol Endocrinol* 1: 816–822

132 Mason SA, Housley PR (1993) Site-directed mutagenesis of the phosphorylation sites in the mouse glucocorticoid receptor. *J Biol Chem* 268: 21501–21504

133 Almlof T, Wright APH, Gustafsson J-A (1995) Role of acidic and phosphorylated residues in gene activation by the glucocorticoid receptor. *J Biol Chem* 270: 17535–17540

134 Hu JM, Bodwell JE, Munck A (1994) Cell cycle-dependent glucocorticoid receptor phosphorylation and activity. *Mol Endocrinol* 8: 1709–1713

135 Oakley RH, Jewell CM, Yudt MR, Bofetiado DM, Cidlowski JA (1999) The dominant negative activity of the human glucocorticoid receptor beta isoform: specificity and mechanisms of action. *J Biol Chem* 274: 27857–27866

136 Leung DYM, Hamid Q, Vottero A, Szefler SJ, Surs W, Minshall E, Chrousos GP, Klemm DJ (1997) Association of glucocorticoid insensitivity with increased expression of glucocorticoid receptor β. *J Exp Med* 186: 1567–1574

137 Shahidi H, Vottero A, Stratakis CA, Taymans SE, Karl M, Longui CA, Chrousos GP, Daughaday WH, Gregory SA, Plate JMD (1999) Imbalanced expression of the glucocorticoid receptor isoforms in cultured lymphocytes from a patient with systemic glucocorticoid resistance and chronic lymphocytic leukemia. *Biochem Biophys Res Commun* 254: 559–565

138 Bronnegard M, Carlstedt-Duke J (1995) The genetic basis of glucocorticoid resistance. *Trends Endocrinol Metab* 6: 160–164

139 Hurley DM, Accili D, Stratikis CA, Karl M, Vamvakopoulos N, Rorer E, Constantine K, Taylor SI, Chrousos GP (1991) Point mutation causing a single amino acid substitution in the hormone binding domain of the glucocorticoid receptor in familial glucocorticoid resistance. *J Clin Invest* 87: 680–686

140 Malchoff C, Brufsky A, Reardon G, McDermott P, Javier E, Bergh CH, Rowe D, Malchoff C (1993) A mutation of the glucocorticoid receptor in primary cortisol resistance. *J Clin Invest* 91: 1918–1924

141 Moalli PA, Pillay S, Krett NL, Rosen ST (1993) Alternatively spliced glucocorticoid receptor messenger RNAs in glucocorticoid-resistant human multiple myeloma cells. *Cancer Res* 53: 3877–3879

142 Strasser-Wozak EMC, Hattmannstorfer R, Hala M, Hartmann BL, Fiegl M, Geley S, Kofler R (1995) Splice site mutation in the glucocorticoid receptor gene causes resistance to glucocorticoid-induced apoptosis in a human acute leukemic cell line. *Cancer Res* 55: 348–353

143 Gaitan D, DeBold CR, Turney MK, Zhou P, Orth DN, Kovacs WJ (1995) Glucocorticoid receptor structure and function in an adrenocorticotropin-secreting small cell lung cancer. *Mol Endocrinol* 9: 1193–1201

144 Bresnick EH, Dalman FC, Sanchez ER, Pratt WB (1989) Evidence that the 90 kDa heat shock protein is necessary for the steroid binding conformation of the L cell glucocorticoid receptor. *J Biol Chem* 264: 4992–4997

145 Nemoto T, Ohara-Nemoto Y, Denis M, Gustafsson JA (1990) The transformed glucocorticosteroid receptor has a lower steroid-binding affinity than the nontransformed receptor. *Biochemistry* 29: 1880–1886

146 Picard D, Khursheed B, Garabedian MJ, Fortin MG, Lindquist S, Yamamoto KR (1990) Reduced levels of hsp90 compromise steroid receptor action *in vivo*. *Nature* 348: 166–168

147 Cadepond F, Binart N, Chambraud B, Jibard N, Schweizer-Groyer G, Segard-Maurel I, Baulieu EE (1993) Interaction of glucocorticosteroid receptor and wild-type or mutated 90-kDa heat shock protein coexpressed in baculovirus-infected Sf9 cells. *Proc Natl Acad Sci USA* 90: 10434–10438

148 Cadepond F, Jibard N, Binart N, Schweizer-Groyer G, Segard-Maurel I, Baulieu EE (1994) Selective deletions in the 90 kDa heat shock protein (hsp90) impede hetero-oligomeric complex formation with the glucocorticosteroid receptor (GR) or hormone binding by GR. *J Steroid Biochem Mol Biol* 48: 361–367

149 Whitesell L, Cook P (1996) Stable and specific binding of heat shock protein 90 by geldanamycin disrupts glucocorticoid receptor function in intact cells. *Mol Endocrinol* 10: 705–712

150 Ning Y-M, Sanchez ER (1993) Potentiation of glucocorticoid receptor-mediated gene expression by the immunophilin ligands FK506 and rapamycin. *J Biol Chem* 268: 6073–6076

151 Ning Y-M, Sanchez ER (1995) Stabilization *in vitro* of the untransformed glucocorticoid receptor complex of S49 lymphocytes by the immunophilin ligand FK506. *J Steroid Biochem Mol Biol* 52: 187–194

152 Allgood VE, Powell-Oliver FE, Cidlowski JA (1990) The influence of vitamin B_6 on the structure and function of the glucocorticoid receptor. *Ann N Y Acad Sci* 585: 452–465

153 Allgood VE, Powell-Oliver FE, Cidlowski JA (1990) Vitamin B_6 influences glucocorticoid receptor-dependent gene expression. *J Biol Chem* 265: 12424–12433

154 Allgood VE, Cidlowski JA (1992) Vitamin B_6 modulates transcriptional activation by multiple members of the steroid hormone receptor superfamily. *J Biol Chem* 267: 3819–3824

155 Allgood VE, Oakley RH, Cidlowski JA (1993) Modulation by vitamin B_6 of glucocorticoid receptor-mediated gene expression requires transcription factors in addition to the glucocorticoid receptor. *J Biol Chem* 268: 20870–20876

156 Burns K, Duggan B, Atkinson EA, Famulski KS, Nemer M, Bleackley RC, Michalak M (1994) Modulation of gene expression by calreticulin binding to the glucocorticoid receptor. *Nature* 367: 476–480

157 Dedhar S, Rennie PS, Shago M, Hagesteijn C-Y, Yang H, Filmus J, Hawley RG, Bruchovsky N, Cheng H, Matusik RJ, Giguere V (1994) Inhibition of nuclear hormone receptor activity by calreticulin. *Nature* 367: 480–483

158 Wheeler DG, Horsford J, Michalak M, White JH, Hendy GN (1995) Calreticulin inhibits vitamin D3 signal transduction. *Nucl Acid Res* 23: 3268–3274

159 Michalak M, Burns K, Andrin C, Mesaeli N, Jass GH, Busaan JL, Opas M (1996) Endoplasmic reticulum form of calreticulin modulates glucocorticoid-sensitive gene expression. *J Biol Chem* 271: 29436–29445

Molecular and cellular aspects of cytokine regulation by glucocorticoids

Fotini Paliogianni[1] and Dimitrios T. Boumpas[2]

[1] *Department of Microbiology, University of Patra, Patra 26224 Greece*
[2] *National Institutes of Health, Bethesda, Maryland 20892, USA; and Division of Rheumatology Clinical Immunology and Allergy, University of Crete, Heraklion 71300, Greece*

Introduction

Glucocorticoids (GC) are potent immunosuppressive agents that have been successfully used in the management of several disorders associated with heightened immunity including transplant rejection, autoimmune diseases and inflammatory disorders [1]. Lymphocytes and macrophages, as primary effectors of cellular and humoral immune responses, are the main targets of their immunoregulatory action [2–10].

Activated T-cells and macrophages produce cytokines. Cytokines are local and systemic protein mediators known to be involved in inflammation, and immunity. The central role of cytokines in immunocyte cross-talk, activation and recruitment favors cytokine inhibition as the major immunosuppressive mechanism of GC action (Tab. 1).

This chapter describes our evolving understanding of the effects of GC on cytokines of the immune system and the mechanisms involved. Cytokines produced by a variety of non-immune cells such as endothelial cells, fibroblasts, keratinocytes, osteoblasts and other cells, are also affected by GC and the mechanisms discussed here are applicable to them as well.

Effects on T-cell activation: an overview

Early activation events

T-lymphocyte activation is controlled by the T-cell antigen receptor (TCR) in combination with signals triggered by accessory molecules present on the surface of the antigen presenting cells (APC). A second group of stimuli required to initiate the pathway of differentiation are the secreted products of macrophages such as IL-1 and/or IL-6. This can be replaced at least in part by phorbol esters that activate protein kinase C (PKC). Binding of antigen to the

Table 1. Cytokine gene modulation by glucocorticoids[1]

Cytokine	Cell type	Effect	Mechanism of action
IL-1α	Peritoneal macrophages, monocytic cell lines	↓	GRE binding, posttranscriptional
IL-1β	Human monocytes promonocytic cell lines	↓	GRE binding, (negative GRE) posttranscriptional
IL-2	T-cells	↓	Tranascription factor antagonism, posttranscriptional
IL-3	Helper T-cell lines	↓	Posttranscriptional
IL-4	T-cells	↑	Transcriptional, no GRE involved
IL-5	T-cells	↓	Unknown
IL-6	T-cells, macrophages, monocytic cell lines	↓	Transcription factor antagonism, GRE binding
IL-8	Epithelial cells, fibroblasts	↓	GRE binding, transcription factor antagonism, posttranscriptional
IL-10	Human monocytes	↑	Unknown
IL-12	T-cells, monocytes monocytic cell lines	↓	Unknown
IL-13	T-cells	↑	Unknown
IFN-γ	T-cells	↓	GRE binding, posttranscriptional
TNF-α	Macrophages, monocytic cell lines	↓	GRE binding, transcription factor antagonism
TGF-β	T-cells, fibroblasts	↑	Transcriptional, posttranscriptional

[1] GRE, glucocorticoid responsive element.

TCR initiates a cascade of events including phosphorylations of intracellular proteins on tyrosine residues and the production of the second messengers Ca^{2+} and diacyl glycerol (Fig. 1). Ca^{2+} binds to and activates its intracellular receptor calmodulin (CAM), which in turn activates CAM-dependent protein kinases and phosphatases, whereas diacylglycerol activates protein kinase C (PKC) (reviewed in [11]). Signal requirements for cytokine production differ; for example signals generated by increased Ca^{2+} concentration and activation of PKC are required for IL-2 production, whereas Ca^{2+} mediated signals are both essential and sufficient for IL-4 production.

Recent studies have established that the Ca^{2+}/calmodulin-dependent protein kinase II (CaM-Kinase II) is a general or multifunctional kinase of Ca^{2+} signaling systems [12]. Following an increase in intracellular free Ca^{2+} concentration, Ca^{2+}/calmodulin activates Cam-Kinase II which phosphorylates itself on the Thr^{286} site of the autoinhibitory domain. This phosphorylation results in inactivation of the autoinhibitory domain that produces a Ca^{2+} independent from of kinase with approximately 20 to 80% of maximal Ca^{2+} stimulated activity [13]. Increase in Ca^{2+} concentration and activation of calmodulin may

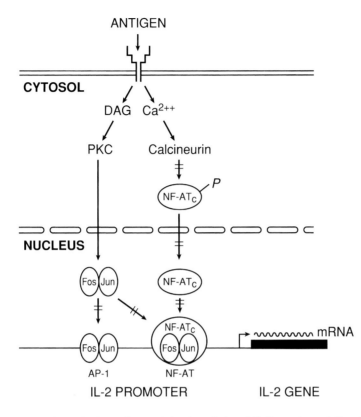

Figure 1. Signal transduction and transcriptional regulation of IL-2 gene transcription sites of GC inhibition are represented with two horizontal bars in this figure. Binding of antigen to the T-cell antigen receptor produces the second messengers diacylglycerol (DAG) and calcium (Ca^{2+}). DAG stimulates PKC which activates the binding of the nuclear proteins Fos and Jun to the AP-1 site of the IL-2 promoter. Ca^{2+} activates calcineurin which dephosphosphorylates NF-ATc. NF-ATc migrates and binds to the NF-AT site within the nucleus along with the Fos and Jun heterodimer. Binding of these nuclear factors and others not shown here (NF-κB, OCT-1) initiates IL-2 gene transcription and production of mRNA. GCR physically interacts with the Fos/Jun heterodimer and inhibits its binding to the AP-1 site and (likely) its association with NF-AT. In addition, GC may inhibit calcineurin-dependent pathways for NF-AT activation.

also activate Ca^{2+}/calmodulin-dependent phosphatases such as calcineurin, a key enzyme for cytokine gene transcription [14]. Calcineurin is the gatekeeper enzyme for IL-2 gene transcription and can separately lead to the transactivation of nuclear factors NFAT, OCT-1, NF-κB [15]. TCR regulated tyrosine kinases induce inositol phospholipid breakdown generating PKC and calcineurin signals, and activate Ras signaling pathways.

Ras pathways serve to link membrane receptors with downstream kinases including the mitogen activated protein kinase cascades. Ras is activated both as a result of PKC-mediated inhibition of Ras-GTPase activating proteins and by an additional signal that is independent of PKC. In the GTP-bound state,

Ras stimulates the MAP kinase pathway consisting of ERK1 and ERK2. At the plasma membrane active Ras activates protein kinase Raf-1 which phosphorylates and activates the MAP kinase/ERK kinases, MEK 1 and MEK 2, which in turn phosphorylate and activate ERKs. The ultimate importance of these pathways is that they stimulate the expression of genes encoding proteins for T-cell effector function and clonal expansion. This is accomplished in large part by the activation of transcription factors that bind to regulatory regions of cytokine genes and thereby enhance promoter activity and transcription of T-cell genes. Ras and Raf activities are required for IL-2 gene expression; MEK-1 and Raf-1 enhance NF-AT driven transcription [16].

GC has profound effects on early activation events following TCR triggered signaling. A selective effect on tyrosine phosphorylation is the inhibition of proteins of 100 KD only in response to TCR activation, but not after stimulation of T-cells with anti-CD2 [3]. Thus, it appears that the effect of GC on tyrosine phosphorylation is signal specific. The nature of this protein has not yet been identified, but it could be the valosin containing protein (VCP), the mammalian analogue of cdc16. Although GC do not have any effect on Ca^{2+} flux *per se*, they have a significant impact on enzymes regulated by activated Ca^{2+}-calmodulin complex. Thus, GC at both pharmacologic and near-physiologic dose, regulate Cam kinase II activity by induction of protein phosphatase activity and abrogation of Cam kinase II autophosphorylation. Inhibition by GC requires at least 6 h preincubation and is fully reversed by RU 486, suggesting that it involves new protein synthesis and is mediated through the GCR [17]. Cam kinase II is a key enzyme regulating the activity of transcription factors involved the cytokine gene transcription in T-cells [18].

As mentioned above, the "gatekeeper" enzyme for T-cell activation and gene transcription is calcineurin. Immunosuppressant CSA and FK506, which interfere with cytokine gene transcription, directly bind and inactivate calcineurin, thus inhibiting cytokine gene transcription. GC do not directly bind calcineurin, but interfere with calcineurin dependent transactivating pathways (see below). Given that all these activation pathways are interegulated, the effect of GC on two main enzymes of Ca^{2+} dependent pathways renders them key regulators of cytokine gene expression. It is of interest that GC have no effect on translocation of PKC, nor on its kinase activity [17]. The effect of GC on the Ras activation pathway are not known at present.

Transcriptional events

Cytokine gene transcription is governed by the formation of highly cooperative assemblies containing a precise arrangement of many proteins including transcription factors, DNA-binding proteins that facilitate their spatial arrangement, and co-activators that bridge the transcription factors and the basal transcription complex. We will next review transcription factors activated during T-cell activation whose activity is affected directly or indirectly by GC.

Nuclear factor of activated T-cells (NFAT)

Despite their name, NF-AT proteins are expressed exclusively in T-cells and are activated by receptors coupled to calcium mobilization. Receptor stimulation and calcium mobilization results in activation of many intracellular pathways including the calcium and calmodulin-dependent phosphatase calcineurin, a major upstream regulator of NFAT proteins.

At least four NFAT-family proteins (NFATp, NAFATc, NAFAT3, NFAT4/NFATx) have been described. NFATp is expressed at high levels in resting T-cells, whereas NFATc is induced following activation. This suggests that NFATp regulates an early stage, while NFATc a latter stage of cytokine transcription [19]. NFAT involvement is well established for IL-2 and IL-4 cytokine genes in T-cells [20, 21] but not for IL-3, IL-5 and IL-8 [22–24].

Three distinct steps for activation of NF-AT have been defined: dephosphorylation, nuclear translocation and increase in affinity for DNA. In resting T-cells, NFATp proteins reside in cytoplasm, are phosphorylated and show low affinity for DNA. Stimuli that elicit Ca^{2+} mobilization result in rapid dephosphorylation of NFAT proteins and their translocation to the nucleus. Dephosphorylated NF-AT proteins show increased affinity for DNA. NFAT proteins interact directly with calcineurin within the cell. Dephosphorylation by calcineurin at multiple sites in their regulatory domains regulates the nuclear import of NFAT proteins. Additional signaling pathways and proteins other than calcineurin, modulate NFAT function in T-cells. For example, increases in Ca^{2+} concentration lead to activation of other calmodulin-dependent enzymes including the multifunctional Ca^{2+}/calmodulin-dependent kinases (CamK), which also regulates NFAT activity. In Jurkat T-cells where a constitutively active form of T-cell CamK II, partially inhibited both NFAT and AP-1 gene expression [18]. The opposite effect was observed for constitutively active CamK IV/GR [25].

The paradigm of NFAT/AP-1 cooperation has been recognized in a number of different cytokine promoter/enhancer regions including IL-2 [26], IL-4 [27], GM-CSF [28], and IFN-γ [29]. The cooperative binding of these two transcription factors results in a complex that is significantly more stable or of higher affinity than those containing each individual factor alone.

GC do not affect directly NF-AT binding or transactivation. The inhibitory effect is indirect [26] through interference with AP-1 cooperation (Fig. 1; see below).

NFκB

NFκB is a protein complex that enables a large number of genes to be rapidly induced in response to extracellular stimuli. Although first described as a B-cell nuclear factor that bound a site in the immunoglobulin κ enhancer, it was subsequently shown that NF-κB binding sites are present in the promoter of many genes most of which are not B-cell specific. These include among others the cytokine genes IL-2, IL-6, GM-CSF and IL-8 [30].

NFκB is a member of the NFκB Rel family. Five members of the mammalian NFκB/Rel proteins have been identified that are characterized by the Rel homology domain (RHD), an N-terminal region of approximately 300 amino acids. The active DNA binding NFκB is a dimer. Classic NFκB is composed of p50 and p65 (or Rel A) subunits.

In unstimulated cells, the NFκB heterodimer is kept as an inactive cytoplasmic complex by inhibitory proteins of the IκB family (IκBα, IκBβ, IκBγ) as well as the NFκB precursor molecules NFκB1 and NFκB2. Inducer-mediated activation of the immune cell correlates with the hyperphosphorylation of IκBα and its subsequent degradation. Paralleling the loss of IκBα in the cytoplasm is the appearance of NFκB in the nucleus. The kinase(s) responsible for IκB phosphorylation have not seen fully characterized yet. Hyperphosphorylated IκB is attached to ubiquitin and degraded by the cytoplasmic proteasome complex. The IκBα isoform is one of the genes whose transcription is initiated by binding of NFκB so that the degradation of IκBα initiates its own synthesis resulting in a negative feedback [30].

In the nucleus NFκB may interact with other proteins to optimally activate transcription. Interestingly many similarities exist between the NFκB and the NFAT family of proteins. The core sequence of the NFAT recognition site, GGAAAA is very similar to an NFκB half site. NFκB as well as NFAT interacts with members of the Fos/Jun family of proteins [31]. A cooperative interaction between NF-IL-6 and the rel A subunit of NFκB is important in the regulation of GM-CSF gene expression [32]. Signaling through CD28, a costimulatory molecule, also leads to activation and binding of NFκB/Rel forms to a CD28 response element (CD28RE) in IL-2 and IL-3 promoters [33].

The signal transduction pathways involved in controlling activation of NFκB are not fully elucidated. Different inducers initiate their pathways through distinct receptors. How these divergent responses converge on IκB is still unknown. Mutation on Ser 32 and 36 inhibit activation of NFκB controlled by T-cell activation signal or pharmacologic agents such as PMA or okadaic acid (an inhibitor of PP1 and PP2A phosphatases). A single kinase activated by multiple pathways may target these residues in NFκB. Phosphatases play an important role in the activation of NFκB, either by regulating kinase or directly by dephosphorylating IκB. Ca^{2+} dependent phosphatases such as calcineurin, PP1 and PP2A potently activate NFκB, but their specific targets are not known [34].

Glucocorticoids inhibit NFκB by two main mechanisms (Fig. 2). First, the activated GCR directly interacts with and inhibits activated NFκB subunits. A second mechanism involves the transcriptional activation of IκBα gene and increased protein synthesis in response to treatment with glucocorticoids. GC also increase the rate of IκB protein synthesis which in turn traps activated NFκB in inactive cytoplasmic complexes [35–39]. GC are known stimulants of phosphatase activity and phosphatases are clearly involved in NFκB inhibition. Whether stimulation of phosphatase activity by GC mediates some of their inhibitory effects on NFκB is not known at present.

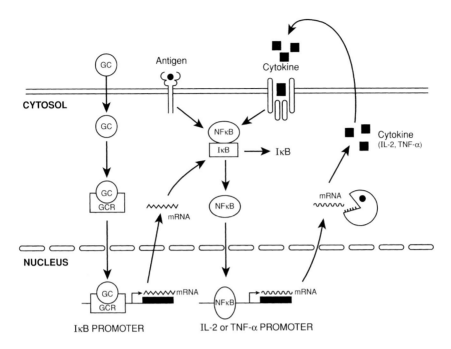

Figure 2. GCR antagonism of NF-κB. Antigen or cytokine binding promotes degradation of the inhibitor κB (IκB) and translocation of NF-κB to the nucleus. GCR either physically interacts with NF-κB preventing its binding to DNA, or stimulates the transcription of NF-κB and the production of additional IκB molecules. This provides a fail-proof mechanism for the inactivation of NF-κB; should any NF-κB molecules escape sequestration by IκB they are rapidly inactivated in the nucleus by associating with GCR. GC also promote the degradation of TNF-α and IL-2 mRNA, and inhibit the translation of TNF-α mRNA. The combination of these effects dramatically decreases the production of TNFα and IL-2.

OCT binding factors

The octamer binding transcription factors OCT-1 and OCT-2 are involved in a wide variety of cellular responses. Originally described as regulators of "housekeeping" genes, these factors were subsequently shown to contribute to inducible transcription. Their action depends on cooperation with other proteins since they lack a strong transcriptional activation domain [40]. Inducible gene expression mediated by OCT protein complex has been shown for cell cycle and viral proteins, early genes and cytokine genes IL-2, 1L-4, and IL-5 [41, 42]. OCT-proteins (NF-IL-2A, OAP/OCT-1 complex) bind a proximal octamer motif on IL-2 promoter that confers responsiveness to signals initiated by the antigen receptor [43]. OCT-1/2 proteins synergize with members of Jun family protein (JunD and c-Jun) [40]. Indirect data suggest that GC inhibit OCT-1 mediated transcription through a mechanism which involves calcineurin dependent pathways [44].

AP-1

Activator protein-1 (AP-1) is a complex transcription factor consisting of Jun and Fos family proteins. AP-1 is activated *via* PKC and by a variety of cytokines (including TNF-α and IL-1β) *via* several types of protein tyrosine kinases and mitogen -activated protein (MAP) kinases. Certain stimuli rapidly increase the transcription of the c-fos gene resulting in increased synthesis of c-fos protein. Other signals lead to activation of kinases that phosphorylate c-jun, resulting in increased activation. For maximal activation of c-jun both phosphorylation and dephosphorylation must occur in different regions of the protein [45]. T-cell activation is in part mediated by the induction of a Jun/AP-1 which leads to the induction of a variety of target genes including cytokines and their receptors [46, 47]. Cross-talk between AP-1 and other transcription factors affecting gene transcription has been clearly established. The inhibitory effect of GC on cytokines involves the functional antagonism between AP-1 and GCR, a model which is described in more details later in this chapter.

Mechanisms of repression of cytokine gene transcription

Similar to other steroids, GC exert their immunoregulatory effects by binding their intracellular receptor, which in turn directly regulates the transcriptional rate of multiple genes (see previous chapters).

Modes of transcriptional repression by GC

CIS -acting effects
These involve protein-DNA interactions. The positive action is exerted by the ligand-induced activation of the GCR. The activated GCR migrates then to the nucleus and acts as a transcription factor that binds directly to a cis-acting sequence (the GRE). This binding is essential for increased gene expression. In essence, GRE functions as inducible enhancer element. GCR has also been shown to repress expression of a variety of genes including cytokine genes; repression of these genes is mediated by binding of the GCR to other DNA regulatory sequences termed negative GRE; alternatively binding to GRE may also displace other transcriptional activators essential for their transcription [48–56].

That GC alter transcription by binding of the activated GCR to GRE is supported by several findings. First, resistance to GC is associated with significant reduction in the capacity of GCR to bind GRE largely stemming from a reduction in GCR numbers. Second, deletion or mutation of either half of the palindromic sequences fails to bind GCR and abolishes dexamethasone-mediated inhibition of gene expression. Third, mutations in the DNA binding domain of the GCR blocks its capacity to bind DNA, thus rendering the receptor transcriptionally inactive.

Trans-acting effects

These involve protein to protein interaction between the GCR and other transcription factors. According to this model, a functional antagonism between GCR and transcription factors is responsible for GC inhibition of cytokine gene expression. Direct protein to protein interaction between GCR and the transcription factors prevents binding of the transcription factor to its DNA-binding site. Direct data supporting this model include the following: 1) Direct interaction between GR and the p50/p65 subunits of NFκB; of note, a zinc finger domain of GCR is necessary for interaction with p65 [51]; 2) Direct interaction between GCR and the POU domain of the octamer factors [52]; and 3) Physical interaction between GCR and fos-jun proteins compromising the AP-1 complex [53–55]. Such an association between the GCR with these transcription factors leads to inhibition of IL-2 and IL-6 promoter activity [26, 53–58]. Interactions between GCR and other transcription factors activated by cytokines (STAT5) are discussed elsewhere in this chapter.

Transcriptional respression by GCR may yet involve another mechanism, namely, interaction between the hormone receptor complex and GRE that are in close proximity to responsive elements for other transcription factors. For example, the promoter region of the glycoprotein hormone-a subunit, which is stimulated by cyclic AMP through the cyclic AMP-responsive element, contains a GRE in close proximity; when the receptor dimer binds to its own element it hinders the cyclic AMP-binding protein from exerting its stimulatory effect on that gene [50].

Transcriptional enhancement by GCR has been shown for octamer transcription factors whose cooperative DNA binding with GCR results in synergism *in vitro* [59]. Transcriptional activation correlates closely with a striking increase in the occupancy of octamer motifs adjacent to GREs on transiently transfected DNAs. Hormone-activated GCR can positively modulate the expression of AP-1-dependent genes, depending on the subunits of the dimeric AP-1 complex. This type of regulation does not require the presence of a GCR binding site in the promoter and is mediated through the DNA binding domain of Jun [60].

Given the differences in experimental conditions employed in accessing GC effects (primary cultures *vs* cell lines *vs* transfectants) the proposed models for GC mediated modulation of transcription of different genes are not mutually exclusive. Whether GC inhibit cytokine gene transcription by interfering with protein-DNA or by protein-protein interactions needs further evaluation. On the other hand, differences in the response among cells or cytokines to the inhibitory action of glucocorticoids may be dependent on the relative abundance of transcription factors. (See below under GC resistance)

Post transcriptional repression of cytokine gene expression

Although the primary control of cytokine gene expression occurs at the transcriptional level, posttranscriptional mechanisms also play important roles in cytokine gene regulation. The mRNAs encoding for many inducible cytokines and lymphokines have been cloned and found to share common sequences that are thought to be essential for regulating their turnover and transient expression. Cytoplasmic factors that depend on the state of activation bind to these sequences and are considered to be responsible for selected expression of different cytokines. Sequences that confer mRNA instability are located at the 3-UTR region of mRNA and are rich in AU sequences (AREs) [61, 62]. AREs are loosely defined as the five nucleotide sequence AUUUA embedded in an uracil-rich region.

Cytokine mRNAs rich in AREs have been reported for IL-1,IL-2, IL-10, TNF-α, and GM-CSF. Specific transacting factors that are not present in quiescent T-cells, but are rapidly induced by stimulation of T-cell receptor/CD3 complex, bind to ARE's found in lymphokine mRNA and regulate mRNA metabolism [63]. GC alter the binding of these transacting factors. Their effect does not require active protein synthesis and is abolished in the presence of phosphatase inhibitors, suggesting that they likely modify the action of an already existing cytoplasmic factor [64]. Since (a) GC exert their function through induction of phosphatase activity, and (b) these transacting factors have been identified as phosphoproteins [65], the effect of GC at the posttrascriptional level may be partly mediated by ARE binding proteins.

The proposed mechanism for GC's mediated mRNA instability through the 3-UTR region of mRNA is not the only one. Thus, in other cells or cell lines the mRNA destabilization effect requires *de novo* mRNA and protein synthesis suggesting that a GC-inducible protein, probably an endonuclease, might influence the stability of a specific mRNA. This mechanism has been shown to be involved in mediating the effects of GC on the IL-1β gene [66].

GC may also alter translational or posttranslational events such as protein stability, processing or secretion. Direct binding of GCR to tRNA [67] may contribute to the translational effects of GG; however other mechanisms have also been implicated. For example, members of AU-binding proteins belong to a heterogenous nuclear ribonucleoprotein hnRNP protein family and are involved in the transfer of mRNA from the nucleus to the cytoplasm [68]. Although no direct data exist thus far to support this, they could represent an additional site for the action of GC. Finally, interaction with JUN-terminal kinase/stress activated protein kinase (JNK/SAPK) has been shown to be involved in mediating inhibition of TNF-a translation by GC [10].

In light of the multiplicity of GC's effects coupled with the differential requirements for induction of cytokine genes in different cell types, a single mechanism may not account for all posttranscriptional effects of GC. Differenct mechanisms may be operant depending upon the cell type, the stimulus and/or the status of activation of cells.

Modulation of cytokine receptors by glucocorticoids

Cytokines exert pleiotropic and redundant functions *via* their receptors expressed on multiple target cells. The reciprocal interaction between cytokines and their receptors represents a complex web that regulates the production of cytokines and their action on target cells. Cytokines can be divided to Type I and Type II cytokines. Type I cytokines comprise the α-helical cytokines that bind to Type I receptors and include interleukins and colony-stimulating factors (Tab. 2). Closely related are the receptors for the interferons (Type II cytokine receptors). This superfamily can be further divided into subgroups based on the use of shared subunits. Sharing of subunits by cytokine receptors provides a molecular explanation for the redundant nature of cytokines [69, 70].

Multiple pathways are involved in tranducing extracellular signals into the nucleus (reviewed in [71]). Once such pathway, the JAK-STAT pathway, involves a novel mechanism in which cytosolic latent transcription factors known as signal transducers and activators of transcription (STATs) are tyrosine phosphorylated by Janus family tyrosine kinases (JAKs) allowing STAT protein dimerization and nuclear translocation. STATs then can modulate the expression of the target genes (Fig. 3).

Table 2. Cytokine-activated Jaks and STATs (Modified from ref. [71])

	Jaks	STATs
Type I Cytokines		
– Cytokines whose receptors share γ_C		
IL-2, IL-7, IL-9, IL-15	Jak1, Jak3	Stat5a, Stat5b, Stat3
IL-4	Jak1, Jak3	Stat6
IL-13*	Jak1, Jak2, Tyk2	Stat6
– Cytokines whose receptors share β_C		
IL-3, IL-5, GM-CSF	Jak2	Stat5a, Stat5b
– Cytokines whose receptors share gp130		
IL6, IL-11	Jak1, Jak2, Tyk2	Stat3
IL-12+	Jak2, Tyk2	Stat4
Type II Cytokines		
– Interferons		
IFNα, IFNβ	Jak1, Tyk2	Stat1, Stat2
IFNγ	Jak1, Jak2	Stat1
IL-10±	Jak1, Tyk2	Stat3

* IL-13 does not share γ_C, but uses IL-4Rα.
+ IL-12 does not share gp130, but it receptor is related to gp130.
± IL-10 is not an interferon, but its receptor is a type II cytokine receptor.

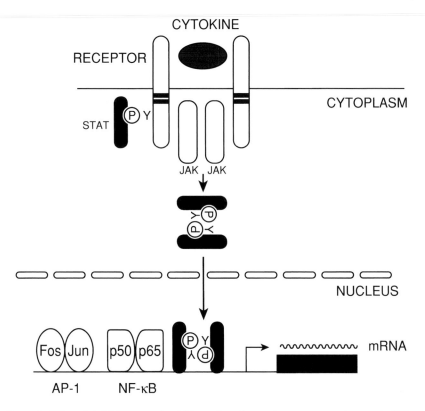

Figure 3. GC mediated inhibition of cytokine action. Among immunosuppressive agents GC are unique since they inhibit both the production (see Figs 1 and 2) and action of proinflammatory cytokines. Binding of cytokines to their receptors stimulates a variety of transcription factors including AP-1, NF-κB and STATs. Activation of STATs occurs through transphosphorylation with JAKs which leads to dimerization with anothr STAT molecule. Dimerized STATs migrate into the nucleus and promote gene transcription. GCR physically interact with AP-1, NF-κB and STATs inhibiting their binding to DNA and transcription of genes. On the other hand, upregulation of these nuclear factors may antagonize the effects of GC promoting GC resistance.

GC have diverse effects on cytokine receptors that parallels their effects on local and systemic inflammatory responses. Although in general GC decrease the level of cytokines in the peripheral blood, they have diverse effects on cytokine receptors including both upregulation and downregulation. Thus, it has been recognized by several groups that GC upregulate the IL-1 R type 1and 2 in different cell types stimulated with a variety of stimuli [72, 73]. The main level of control is posttranscriptional. The same effect has been described for IL-6 [74, 75], GM-CSF [76] and IFN-γ receptors [77, 78]. Although GC clearly upregulate receptor density on target cells, they have no effect on the binding affinity of receptors to their ligands [75, 78]. The IL-10 receptor is also upregulated by GC in human keratinocytes [79]. IL-10 is overexpressed in atopic dermatitis while its receptor is dramatically decreased in acute exanthematic psoriatic epidermis. Upregulation of IL-10R by GC could explain their beneficial effect in antipsoriatic therapy [79].

Whereas GC clearly up-regulate proinflammatory cytokine receptors their effects on the TNF receptors are inhibitory. GC inhibit the release of soluble TNF receptors by human monocytes concurrenly with suppression of TNF-α production [80]. In human airway epithelial cells GC increase the total cellular 55kd TNF type 1 receptor, but inhibit its release in soluble forms [81].

The effect of GC on IL-2 receptor expression remains controversial. In primary human lymphocytes stimulated by mitogens IL-2Ra expression has been shown to be both upregulated [82] by GC and inhibited [83]. IL-2 induced expression of IL-2Ra in activated T-cells is also inhibited by GC while exogenous IL-2 overcomes the GC mediated inhibition [83]. The inhibitory effect of GC on IL-2R expression is probably indirect and resulting from decreased IL-2 production and inhibition of NF-κB binding [6, 83–85].

IL-4 and IL-5 receptor expression is inhibited by GC *in vitro* and *in vivo* [86, 87]. Their effect is mainly posttranscriptional and could account for GC's beneficial effects in certain allergic diseases where these receptors are upregulated.

GC effects on STATs are only now beginning to be understood. STAT5 is tyrosine phosphorylated by Janus protein tyrosine kinases which subsequently interact with the SH2 domain of its dimerization partner and binds to DNA at STAT-response elements to induce transcription. STAT5 is activated in response to a variety of cytokins including IL-2, IL-3, IL-5, IL-7, IL-9, IL-15 and GM-CSF (Tab. 2). STAT5 forms a complex with the GR which binds to DNA independently of the GRE. Formation of this complex between STAT5 and the GR diminishes the glucocorticoid response of a GRE containing promoter [88]. GC are known to synergistically enhance IL-6 mediated cellular responses. STAT3, a transcriptional factor activated among others, by IL-6, can associate with and synergize with the GR to increase transcription of IL-6 inducible genes [89, 90].

Effect of GC on TH1/TH2 orientation

T-helper lymphocytes can be divided into two distinct subsets of effector cells based on their functional capabilities and the profile of cytokines they produce. The Th1 subset secretes IL-2, IFN-γ and TNF-α and induces cell mediated immune responses; Th2 cells produce cytokines such as IL-4, IL-5 IL-10 and IL-13 that are associated with humoral immune responses. The selective differentiation of either subset is established during priming and can be significantly influenced by a variety of factors. One of these factors, the cytokine environment, has been established as the major variable influencing Th development [91]. Defense against infectious microorganisms, allergic reactions, autoimmune responses and allograft rejections are regulated by Th1/Th2 balance of cytokines produced during the course of immune response.

Glucocorticoids have opposing immunoregulatory effects on the Th1/Th2 responses; they suppress the production of Th1 type cytokines such as IL-2, IL-12, IFN-γ and TNF-α while augmenting the production Th2 cytokines such as IL-4, IL-10, and IL-13, both *in vivo* and *in vitro* [92–97]. GC also down-regulate the transcriptional activity of the IL-2 promoter, but upregulate that of the IL-4 promoter [98]. In experimental allergic encephalomyelitis (EAE) in Lewis rats (a cell mediated autoimmune disease induced by Th1 T cells in response to myelin basic protein) plasma levels of GC are elevated during spontaneous recovery. In these animals adrenalectomy leads to progressive disease which can be reversed by GC replacement [99]. It has been suggested that GC contribute to the compensatory shift from a Th1 to a Th2 response thus facilitating recovery from this disease.

In humans, elevated plasma GC during the stress response induces a shift toward a Th2 cytokine response [100], suggesting that under physiological conditions endogenous GC may polarize the immune response towards the Th2 direction. Although GC may affect cytokine production and Th1/Th2 polarization of T-cells in several ways, the primary mechanism underlying the shift to Th2 response is inhibition of IL-12 by macrophages [101]. IL-12 is extremely potent in inhibiting IL-4 and enhancing IFN-γ synthesis in both unprimed as well as resting cells [102]. GC also enhance IL-10 production in human peripheral monocytes [100, 103, 104]. Inhibition of IL-12 paralleled with increased IL-10 production may account for IL-4 production and shift to Th2 response. Another possible mechanism in animals is the enhancement of survival of NK1.1$^+$ T cells [105]. NK1.1$^+$ T-cells are considered to influence the commitment towards the Th1/Th2 lineage, because they promptly produce IL-4 after stimulation with anti-CD3 mAb.

GC resistance and cytokines

The efficacy of GC therapy in a variety of chronic immune mediated diseases is unpredictable. Clinical and laboratory evidence suggest that patients can be divided into GC-sensitive and GC-resistant groups. These differences have been documented in the treatment of asthma, rheumatoid athritis and in renal graft recipients [106–116]. This resistance may be hereditary due to mutations in the GCR gene detected by PCR-based techniques (estimated to be present in ~2.3% of the normal population), or acquired as is the case of patients with hematologic malignancies and autoinflammatory diseases. On the other hand, other abnormalities in the GCR may render ~6.6% of the normal population relatively hypersensitive to GC [106].

Several mechanisms have been implicated in GC resistance [117]. Alternative splicing of the GCR pre-mRNA generates a second receptor, named GCR-beta, which does not bind GC, but antagonizes the transactivating activity of the classic GCR, GCR-alpha [118–120]. Patients with GC-insensitive asthma have higher numbers of GCR-beta immunoreactive cells in peripheral blood [120] and cytokine-induced abnormalities in the DNA binding of the GCR [121]. A variety of cytokines (IL-1, IL-2, IL-6, IFN-γ) seem to abrogate the GC mediated inhibition of T-cells proliferation [122]. IL-2 and IL-4 may reduce the binding affinity of GCR which may contribute to the development of GC-resistance and persistent inflammation [117, 123]. Other potential mechanisms for cytokine mediated GC resistance include interactions of GCR with cytokine induced transcription factors such as AP-1, NF-κB and STAT5 inhibiting its activity. IL-1α inhibits GCR translocation and hormone-induced GCR-mediated gene transcription and may also promote GC resistance [109].

Concluding remarks and future directions

In addition to their salutary effects on the treatment of inflammatory diseases, GC have also been proven to be useful tools to dissect signal transduction and cytokine pathways in the immune system. *In vitro* systems, although useful in establishing mechanisms of action, are rather artificial and limited for us to be able to interpret *in vivo* scenarios in humans. To overcome these problems investigators have begun to use more reliable *in vivo* systems such as human-animal chimeras [124]. Given the extensive interactions among various cytokines the effect of GC may be more widespread and not necessarily limited to a few cytokines.

For the future, we need better methods to predict clinical responsiveness to GC (and its mechanisms) in combination with less toxic, but equally efficacious compounds. To this end, synthetic GC have been developed that dissociate transactivation and AP-1 transexpression. These compounds retain the anti-inflammatory and immunosuppressive potential of classic GC, but have weak transactivating effects on genes involved in neoglycogenesis and the GC-associated side-effects [125].

References

1 Boumpas DT, Chrousos GP, Wilder RL, Cupps TR, Balow JE (1993) Glucocorticoid therapy for immune-mediated diseases: basic and clinical correlates. *Ann Intern Med* 119: 1198–1208

2 Boumpas DT, Paliogianni F, Anastassiou ED, Balow (1991) Glucocorticosteroid action on the immune system: molecular and cellular aspects. *Clin Exp Rheumatol* 9: 413–423

3 Paliogianni F, Ahuja SS, Yamada H, Balow JP, Boumpas DT (1992) Glucocorticoids inhibit T cell proliferation by downregulating proliferative signals mediated through both T cell antigen and interleukin-2 receptors. *Arthritis Rheum* 35: S127 (Abstract)

4 Vacca A, Screpanti I, Maroder M, Felli MP, Farina AR, Gismondi A, Santoni A, Fracti A, Gulino A (1990) Transcriptional regulation of the interleukin-2 gene by glucocorticoid hormones. *J Biol Chem* 265: 8075–8080

5 Adcock IM, Brown CR, Gelder CM, Shirasaki H, Peters MJ, Barnes PJ (1995) Effects of glucocorticoids on transcription factor activation in human peripheral blood mononuclear cell. *Amer J Physiol* 268 (2pt 1): C331–338

6 Paliogianni F, Ahuja SS, Balow JP, Boumpas DT (1993) Novel mechanism for inhibition of human T cells by glucocorticoids (GC): GC modulate signal transduction through IL-2 receptor. *J Immunol* 151: 4081–4089

7 Bowen DL, Fauci AS (1988) Adrenal corticosteroids. *In*: JI Gallin, IM Goldstein, R Snyderman (eds): *Inflammation: basic and clinical correlates*. Haven Press, New York, 935–946

8 Amano Y, Lee SW, Allison AC (1993) Inhibition by glucocorticoids of the formation of interleukin-1a, interkeukin-1β, and interleukin-6: mediation by decrease mRNA stability. *Mol Pharmacol* 43: 176–182

9 Lee SW, Tsuo AP, Chan H, Thomas J, Petrick Eugui EM, Allison AC (1988) Glucocorticoids selectively inhibit the transcription of the interleukin-1β gene and decrease the stability of interleukin 1β mRNA. *Proc Natl Acad Sci USA* 85: 1204–1208

10 Swantek JL, Cobb MH, Geppert TD (1997) Jun N-terminal kinase/stress-activated protein kinase (JNP/SAPK) is required for lipopolysaccaride stimulation of tumor necrosis factor alpha (TNF-α) translation: glucocorticoids inhibit TNF-alpha translation by blocking JNP/SAPK. *Mol Cell Biol* 17: 6274–6282

11 Siegel JN, June CH (1993) Signal transduction in T-cell activation and tolerance. *In*: S Gupta, C Griscelli (eds): *New concepts in immunodeficiency diseases*. John Wiley and Sons, Philadelphia, 85–129

12 Hanson PI, Shulman H (1992) Neuronal Ca^{2+}/calmodulin-dependent protein kinases. *Annu Rev Biochem* 61: 559–601

13 Lou LL, Llyod SJ, Shulman H (1986) Activation of the multifunctional Ca^{2+}/calmodulin protein kinase by autophosphorylation: ATP modulates production of an autonomous enzyme. *Proc Natl Acad Sci USA* 83: 9497–9501

14 Clipstone NA, Crabtree GR (1992) Identification of calcineurin as a key signaling enzyme in T-lymphocyte activation. *Nature* 357: 695–697

15 Emmel EA, Verweij CL, Durand DB, Higgins CM, Lacy E, Crabtree GR (1989) Cyclosporin A specifically inhibits function of nuclear proteins involved in T cell activation. *Science* 246: 1617–1620

16 Cantrell D (1996) T cell antigen receptor signal tranduction pathways. *Annu Rev Immunol* 14: 259–274

17 Paliogianni F, Hama N, Balow JE, Valentine MA, Boumpas DT (1995) Glucocorticoid-mediated regulation of protein phosphorylation in primary human T cells: Evidence for induction of phosphatase activity. *J Immunol* 1809–1817

18 Hama N, Paliogianni F, Fessler BJ, Boumpas DT (1995) Calcium/calmodulin-dependent protein kinase II downregulates both calcineurin and protein kinase C mediated pathways for cytokine gene transcription in human T cells. *J Exp Med* 181: 1217–1222

19 Rao A, Hogan PG (1997) Transcription factors of the NFAT family: Regulation and function. *Annu Rev Immunol* 15: 707–747

20 Jain J, Loh C, Rao A (1995) Transcriptional regulation of the interleukin 2 gene. *Curr Opin Immunol* 7: 333–342

21 Weiss DL, Hural J, Tara D, Timmerman LA, Henkel G, Brown MA (1996) Nuclear factor of activated T cells is associated with a mast cell interleukin 4 transcription complex. *Mol Cell Biol* 16: 228–235

22 Tocci MJ, Matkovich DA, Collier KA, Kwock P, Dumond F, Lin S, Degudicibus S, Siekierka JJ, Chin J, Hutchinson N (1989) The immunosuppressant FK506 selectively inhibits expression of early T activation genes. *J Immunol* 143: 718–726

23 Stranick KS, Payvandi F, Zambas DN, Umland SP, Egan RW, Billah MM (1995) Transcription of the murine interleukin 5 gene is regulated by multiple promoter elements. *J Biol Chem* 270: 20575–20582

24 Okamoto SI, Makaida N, Yasumoto K, Rice N, Ishikawa Y, Horiguchi H, Murakami S, Matsushima K (1994) The interleukin-8 AP1 and κB-like sites are genetic end targets of FK506-sensitive pathway accompanied by calcium mobilization. *J Biol Chem* 269: 8582–8589

25 Ho N, Gullberg M, Chatila T (1996) Activation protein-1 dependent transcriptional activation of interleukin 2 gene by Ca^{2+}/calmodulin kinase type IV/Gr. *J Exp Med* 184: 101–112

26 Paliogianni F, Raptis A, Ahuja SS, Najjar SM, Boumpas DT (1993) Negative transcriptional regulation of human interleukin 2 (1L-2) gene by glucocorticoids through interference with nuclear transcription factors AP-1 and NF-AT. *J Clin Invest* 91: 1481–1489

27 Rooney JW, Hoey T, Glimcher LH (1995) Coordinate and cooperative roles for NFAT and AP-1

in the regulation of the murine IL-4 gene. *Immunity* 2: 473–483

28 Cockerill PN, Bert AG, Jenkins F, Ryan GR, Shannon MF, Vadas MA (1995) Human granulocyte-macrophage colony-stimulating factor enhancer function is associated with cooperative interactions between AP-1 and NFATp/c. *Mol Cell Biol* 15: 2071–2079

29 Campbell PM, Pimm J, Ramassar V, Halloran PF (1996) Identification of calcium-inducible, cyclosporine-sensitive elements in the IFN-γ promoter that is a potential NFAT binding site. *Transplantation* 61: 933–939

30 Albert S, Baldwin Jr, (1996) The NF-κB and IκB proteins: New discoveries and insights. *Annu Rev Immunol* 14: 649–681

31 Schmid R, Liptay S, Betts J, Nabel G (1994) Structural and functional analysis of NF-κB: determinants of DNA binding specificity and protein interaction. *J Biol Chem* 269: 162–167

32 Jain J, Burgeon E, Badalian T, Hogan P, Rao A (1995) A similar DNA-binding motif in NFAT family proteins and the Rel homology region. *J Biol Chem* 270: 4138–4145

33 Ghosh P, Tan TH, Rice N, Sica A, Young H (1993) The IL-2 CD28-responsive complex contains at least three members of the NF-κB family: c-Rel, p50 and p65. *Proc Natl Acad Sci USA* 90: 1696–1700

34 Sun SC, Maggirwar S, Harhaj E (1995) Activation of NF-κB involves the phosphorylation of IkBa at phosphatase 2A-sensitive sites. *J Biol Chem* 270: 3471–3751

35 Auphan N, DiDonato JA, Rosette C, Helmberg A, Karin M (1995) Immunosuppression by glucocorticoids: Inhibition of NF-κB activity through induction of IkB synthesis. *Science* 270: 286–289

36 Scheinman RI, Cogswell PC, Lofquist AK, Baldwin AS (1995) Role of transcriptional activation of IκBα in mediation of immunosuppression by glucocorticoids. *Science* 270: 283–286

37 Ray A, Prefontaine KE (1994) Physical association and functional antagonism between the p65 subunit of transcription factor NF-κB and the glucocorticoid receptor. *Proc Natl Acad Sci USA* 91: 752–756

38 Mukaida N, Morita M, Ishikawa Y, Rice N, Okamoto S, Kasahara T, Matsushima K (1994) Novel Mechanism of glucocorticoid-mediated gene repression. Nuclear factor-κB is target for glucocorticoid-mediated interleukin 8 gene repression. *J Biol Chem* 269: 13289–13295

39 Wissink S, van Heerde EC, vand der Burg B, van der Saag PT (1998) A dual mechanism mediated repression of NF-kappaB activity by glucocorticoids. *Mol Endocrinol* 12: 355–363

40 Ullman KS, Northrop JP, Admon A, Crabtree GR (1993) Jun family members are controlled by a calcium-regulated, cyclosporin A-sensitive signalling pathway in activated T lymphocytes. *Gene Develop* 7: 188–196

41 Gruart-Gouilleux V, Engels P, Sullican M (1995) Characterization of the human interleukin-5 gene promoter: involvement of octamer binding sites in the gene promoter activity. *Eur J Immunol* 25: 1431–1435

42 Pfeuffer I, Klein-Hebling S, Heifling A, Chuvpilo S, Escher C, Brabletz T, Hentsch B, Schwarzenbach H, Matthias P, Serfling E (1994) Octamer factors exert a dual effect on the IL-2 and IL-4 promoter. *J Immunol* 153: 5572–5585

43 Ullman KS, Flanagan WM, Edwards CA, Crabtree GR (1991) Activation of early gene expression in T lymphocytes by Oct-1 and an inducible protein, OAP[40]. *Science* 254: 558–561

44 Paliogianni F, Boumpas DT (1995) Glucocorticoids regulate calcineurin-dependent trans-activating pathways for interleukin-2 gene transcription in human T-lymphocytes. *Transplantation* 59: 1333–1339

45 Currant T, Franza BR (1988) Fos and Jun: the AP-1 connection. *Cell* 55: 395–397

46 Sundstedt A, Sigvardsson M, Leanderson T, Hedlund G, Kalland T, Dohlsten M (1996) *In Vivo* anergized CD4+ T cells express perturbed AP-1 and NK-κB transcription factor. *Proc Natl Acad Sci USA* 93: 979–984

47 Rao A (1994) NF-ATp: a transcription factor required for coordinate induction of several genes. *Immunol Today* 15: 274–281

48 Ray A, LaForge KS, Sehgal PB (1990) On the mechanism for efficient repression of the interleukin-6 promoter by glucocorticoids: enhancer, TATA box, and RNA start site (Inr motif) occlusion. *Mol Cell Biol* 10: 5736–5746

49 Mordacq JC, Linzer DIH (1989) Co-localization of elements required for phorbol ester stimulation and glucocorticoid repression of proliferin gene expression. *Gene Develop* 3: 760–769

50 Akerblom IE, Slater EP, Beato M, Baxter JD, Mellon PL (1988) Negative regulation by glucocorticoids through interference with a cAMP responsive enhancer. *Science* 241: 350–353

51 Ray A, Prefontaine KE (1994) Physical association and functional antagonism between the p65

subunits of transcription factor NF-κB and the glucocorticoid receptor. *Proc Natl Acad Sci USA* 91: 752–756

52 Kutoh E, Stromstedt PE, Poellinger L (1992) Functional interference between the ubiquitous and constitutive octamer transcription factor 1 (OTF-1) and the glucocorticoid receptor by direct protein-protein interaction involving the homeo subdomain of OCT-1. *Mol Cell Biol* 12: 4960–4969

53 Schule R, Rangarajan P, Kliewer S, Ransome LJ, Bolado J, Yank N, Verma IM, Evans RM (1990) Functional antagonism between oncoprotein c-Jun and the glucocorticoid receptor. *Cell* 62: 1217–1226

54 Yang-Yen HF, Chambard JC, Sun YL, Smeal T, Schmidt TJ, Drouin J, Karin M (1990) Transcriptional interference between c-Jun and the glucocorticoid receptor: mutual inhibition of DNA binding due to direct protein- protein interaction. *Cell* 62: 1205–1215

55 Jonat C, Rahmsdorf HJ, Park KK, Cato AC, Gebel S, Ponta H, Herrlich P (1990) Antitumor promotion and antiinflammation: down-modulation of AP-1 (Fos/Jun) activity by glucocorticoid hormone. *Cell* 62: 1189–1204

56 Northrop JP, Crabtree GR, Mattila PS (1992) Negative regulation of interleukin 2 transcription by the glucocorticoid receptor. *J Exp Med* 175: 1235–1245

57 Ray A, LaForge KS, Sehgal PB (1991) Repressor to activator switch by mutations in the first finger of the glucocorticoid receptor: is direct binding necessary? *Proc Natl Acad Sci USA* 88: 7086–7090

58 Nishio Y, Isshiki H, Kishimoto T, Akima S (1993) A nuclear factor for interleukin-6 (NF-IL6) and the glucocorticoid receptor synergistically activate transcription of the rat α1-acid glycoprotein gene *via* direct protein-protein interaction. *Mol Cell Biol* 13: 1854–1862

59 Prefontaine GG, Lemieu ME, Griffin W, Schild-Poulter C, Pope L, LaCasse E, Walker P, Hache RJ (1988) Recruitment of octamer transcription factors to DNA by glucocorticoid receptor. *Mol Cell Biol* 18: 3416–3430

60 Teurich S, Angel P (1995) The glucocorticoid receptor synergizes with Jun homodimers to activate AP-1 regulated promoters lacking GR binding sites. *Chem Senses* 20: 251–255

61 Cleveland DW, Yen JJ (1989) Multiple determinants of eucaryotic mRNA stability. *New Biol* 1: 121–126

62 Kontoyiannis D, Pasparakis M, Pizarro TT, Cominelli F, Kollias G (1999) Impaired on/off regulation of TNF biosynthesis in mice lacking TNF AU-rich elements: implications for joint and gut-associated immunopathologies. *Immunity* 10: 387–398

63 Bohjanen PR, Petryniac B, June CH, Thomson CB, Lindsten T (1991) An inducible cytoplasmic factor (AU-B) binds selectively to AUUA multimers in the 3' untranslated region of lymphokine mRNA. *Mol Cell Biol* 11: 3288–3295

64 Paliogianni F, Balow JE, Boumpas DT (1997) Glucocorticoids modulate the binding of specific proteins to AU-sequences in the 3'-untranslated region (UTR) of interleukin-2 (IL-2) by activating phosphatases 1 and phosphatase 2. *J Alergyl. Clin Immunol* 99: 1954 (Abstract)

65 Matler JS (1989) Identification of an AUUUA-specific messenger RNA binding. *Protein Sci* 246: 664–666

66 Brown EA, Dave HA, Marsh CB, Wewers MD (1996) The combination of endotoxin and dexamethasone induces type II interleukin 1 receptor (IL-1 rII) in monocytes: a comparison to interleukin 1 beta (IL-1 beta) and interleukin 1 receptor antagonist (IL-1ra). *Cytokine* 8: 828–836

67 All M, Vedeckis W (1987) The glucocorticoid receptor protein binds to transfer RNA. *Science* 235: 467–470

68 Katz DA, Theodorakis NG, Cleveland DW, Lindsten T, Thomson CB (1993) AU-A and RNA-binding activity distinct from hnRNA A1, is selective for AUUUA repeats and shuttles between the nucleus and the cytoplasm. *Nucl Acid Res* 22: 238–246

69 O'Shea JJ (1997) Jaks, STATs, cytokine signal transduction and immunoregulation: Are we there yet? *Immunity* 7: 1–11

70 Aringer M, Cheng A, Nelson JW, Chen M, Sudarshan C, Zhou Y-J, O'Shea JJ (1999) Janus kinases and their role in growth disease. *Life Sci* 64: 2173–2186

71 Leonard WJ, O, Shea JJ (1998) JAKs and STATs: Biological implications. *Annu Rev Immunol* 16: 293–322

72 Levine SJ, Benfield T, Shelhamer JH (1996) Corticosteroids induce intracellular interleukin-1 receptor antagonist type I expression by a human airway epithelial cell line. *Amer J Respir Cell Mol Biol* 15: 245–251

73 Ho A, Takii T, Goto N, Kito Y, Onozaki K (1997) Role of glucocorticoid in the upregulation of

type I interleukin-1 receptor mRNA expression in hepatocytes of endotoxin-administrated mice. *J Interferon Cytokine Res* 17: 413–417

74 Pietzko Zohlhofer D, Graeve K Fleischer D, Stoyan T, Schooltink H, Rose-John S, Heinrich PC (1993) The hepatic interleukin-6 receptor. Studies on its structure and regulation by phorbol 12-myristate 13-acetate-dexamethasone. *J Biol Chem* 268: 4250–4258

75 Snyers L, DeWit L, Content J (1990) Glucocorticoid upregulation of high affinity interleukin 6 receptors on human epithelial cells. *Proc Natl Acad Sci USA* 87: 2838–2842

76 Hawrylowicz CM, Guida L, Paleolog E (1994) Dexamethazone upregulates granulocyte-macrophage colony-stimulating factor receptor expression on human monocytes. *Immunology* 83: 274–280

77 Novelli F, Di Pierro F, diCelle PF, Bertini S, Affaticati P, Garotta F, Forni G (1994) Environmental signals influencing expression of the IFN-γ promotes proliferation or apoptosis. *J Immunol* 152: 496–504

78 Strickland RW, Wahl LM, Finbloom DS (1986) Corticosteroids enhance the binding of recombinant interferon-γ to cultured human monocytes. *J Immunol* 137: 1577–1580

79 Michel G, Mirmohammasdadegh A, Olasz E, Jarzeska-Deussen B, Muschen L, Abts HF, Ruzicka T (1997) Demonstration and functional analysis of IL-10 receptors in human epidermal cells: decreased expression in psoriatic skin, down-modulation by IL-8, and up-regulation by an antipsoriatic glucocorticosteroid in normal cultured keratinocytes. *J Immunol* 159: 6291–6297

80 Joyce DA, Kloda A Steer JH (1997) Dexamethasone suppresses release of soluble TNF receptors by human monocytes concurrently with TNF-alpha suppression. *Immun Cell Biol* 75: 345–350

81 Levine SJ, Logun C, Chopra DP, Rhim JS, Shelhamer JH (1996) Protein kinase C, interleukin-1 beta, and corticosteroid regulate shedding of the type I, 55 kDa TNF receptor from human airway epithelial cells. *Amer J Respir Cell Mol Biol* 14: 254–261

82 Lamas M, Sanz E, Martin-Parras L, Espel E, Sperizen P, Collins M, Silva AG (1993) Glucocorticoid hormones upregulate interleukin-2 receptor alpha gene expression. *Cell Immunol* 151: 437–450

83 Boumpas DT, Anastassiou ED, Older SA, Tsokos GC, Nelson DL, Balow JE (1991) Dexamethasone inhibits human interleukin 2 but not interleukin 2 receptor gene expression *in vitro* at the level of nuclear transcription. *J Clin Invest* 87: 1739–1747

84 Wissink S, van Heerde EC, Schmitz ML, Kalkhoven E, van der Burg B, Baeuerle PA, van der Saag PT (1997) Distinct domains of the RelA NK-kappaB subunit are required for negative cross-talk and direct interaction with the glucocorticoid receptor. *J Biol Chem* 272: 22278–22284

85 DeBosscher K, Schmitz ML, Vanden Berghe W, Plaisance S, Fiers W, Haegeman G (1997) Glucocorticoid-mediated repression of nuclear factor-kappaB-dependent transcription involves direct interference with transactivation. *Proc Natl Acad Sci USA* 94: 13504–13509

86 Mozo L, Gayo A, Suarez A, Rivas D, Zamorano J, Gutierrez C (1998) Glucocorticoids inhibit IL-4 and mitogen induced IL-4R alpha chain expression by different posttranscriptional mechanisms. *J Allergy Clin Immunol* 102: 968–976

87 Wright ED, Christodoulopoulos P, Small P, Frenkiel S, Hamid Q (1988) Th-2 type cytokine receptors in allergic rhinitis and in response to topical steroids. *Laryngoscope* 108: 1528–1533

88 Stocklin E, Wissler M, Gouilleux F, Groner B (1996) Functional interactions between Stat5 and the glucocorticoid receptor. *Nature* 383: 726–728

89 Takade T, Kurachi H, Yamamoto T, Nishio Y, Nakatsuji Y, Morishige Ki Miyake A, Murata Y (1998) Crosstalk between the interleukin-6 (IL-6)-JAK-STAT and the glucocorticoid-nuclear receptor pathway; synergistic activation of IL-6 response elements by IL-6 glucocorticoid. *J Endocrinol* 159: 323–330

90 Zhang Z, Jones S, Hagood JS, Fuentes NL, Fuller GM (1997) STAT3 acts as a co-activator of glucocorticoid receptor signaling. *J Biol Chem* 272: 30607–30610

91 Romagnani S (1991) Human Th1 and Th2: doubt no more. *Immunol Today* 12: 256–257

92 Wilder RL (1995) Neuroendocrine-immune system interactions and autoimmunity. *Annu Rev Immunol* 13: 307–338

93 Arya SK, Wong-Staal F, Gallo RC (1984) Dexamethasone-mediated inhibition of human T-cell growth factor and γ-IFN messenger RNA. *J Immunol* 133: 273–276

94 Beutler B, Krochin N, Milsark IW, Luedke C, Cerami A (1986) Control of cachectin (TNF) synthesis: mechanisms of entotoxin resistance. *Science* 232: 977–980

95 Daynes RA, Araneo BA (1989) Contrasting effects of glucocorticoids on the capacity of T cells to produce the growth factors interleukin 2 and interleukin 4. *Eur J Immunol* 19: 2319–2325

96 Ramierz FD, Fowell J, Puklavez M, Simmonds S, Mason D (1996) Glucocorticoids promote a Th2 cytokine response by CD4+ T cells *in vitro. J Immunol* 156: 2406–2412

97 Blotta MH, Dekruyff RH, Umetsu DT (1997) Corticosteroids inhibit IL-12 production in human monocytes and enhance their capacity to induce IL-4 synthesis in CD4+ lymphocytes. *J Immunol* 158: 5589–5595

98 Hama N, Paliogianni F, Mavrothalassitis G, Yamada H, Boumpas DT (1998) Glucorticoid modulation of cytokine gene transcription opposing effects on pro-inflammatory *vs* anti-inflammatory cytokine promoters. *Arthritis Rheum* 41: S194 (Abstract)

99 Macphee IA, Antoni FA, Mason DW (1989) Spontaneous recovery of rats from experimental allergic encephalomyelitis is dependent on regulation of the immune system by endogenous adrenal corticosteroids. *J Exp Med* 169: 431–445

100 Agarwall SK, Marshall GD (1998) Glucocorticoid-induced type 1/type 2 cytokine alterations in humans: a model for stress-related immune disfunction. *J Interferon Cytokine Res* 18: 1059–1068

101 Dekruyff RH, Fang Y, Umetsu TD (1998) Corticosteroids enhance the capacity of macrophages to induce Th2 sytokine sythesis in CD4+ lymphocytes by inhibiting IL-12 production. *J Immunol* 2231–2237

102 Trinchieri G (1995) Interleukin-12: a proinflammatory cytokine with immunoregulatory functions that bridge innate resistance and antigen-specific adaptive immunity. *Annu Rev Immunol* 13: 251–276

103 Visser J, van Boxel-Dezaire A, Methorst D, Brunt T, de Kloet ER, Nagelkerken L (1998) Differential regulation of interleukin 10 (IL-10) and IL-12 by glucocorticoids *in vitro. Blood* 91: 4255–4264

104 Vieira PL, Kalinski P, Wierenga EA, Kapsenberg ML, de Jong EC (1998) Glucocorticoids inhibit bioactive IL-12p70 production by *in vitro* generated human dendritic cells without affecting their T cell stimulatory potential. *J Immunol* 161: 5245–5251

105 Tamada K, Harada M, Koichiro A, Tieli L, Nomoto K (1998) IL-4 producing NK1.1+ T cells are resistant to glucocorticoid-induced apoptosis: Implications for the Th1/Th2 balance. *J. Immunol* 161: 1239–1247

106 Lamberts SWJ, Huizenga ATM, de Lande P, de Jong FH, Koper JW (1996) Clinical aspects of glucocorticoid sensitivity. *Steroids* 61: 157–160

107 Corrigan CJ, Brown PH, Barnes NC, Szefler SJ, Tsia JJ, Frew AJ, Kay AB (1991) Glucocorticoid resistance in chronic asthma. Glurcocorticoid pharmacokinetics, glucocorticoid receptor characteristics, and inhibition of peripheral blood T cell proliferation by glucocorticoids *in vitro. Amer Rev Respir Dis* 144: 1016–1025

108 Morand EF, Jefferiss CM, Dixey J, Mitra D, Goulding NJ (1994) Impaired glucocorticoid induction of mononuclear leukocyte lipocortin-1 in rheumatoid arthritis. *Arthritis Rheum* 37: 207–211

109 Miller AH, Pariante CM, Pearce BD (1996) Effects of cytokines on glucocorticoid receptor expression and function. Glucocorticoid resistanece and relevance to depression. *Adv Exp Med Biol* 461: 107–116

110 Kirkham B, Corkill MM, Davison SC, Panayi GS (1991) Response to glucocorticoid treatment in rheumatoid arthritis: *in vitro* cell mediated immune assay predicts *in vivo* response. *J Rheumatol* 18: 30–33

111 Walker KB, Potter JM, House AK (1985) Variable inhibition of mitogen-induced blastogenesis in human lymphocytes by prednisolone *in vitro. Transplant Proc* 17: 1676–1678

112 Langhoff E, laderfoged J, Jacobsen BK (1986) Reciepient lymphocyte sensitivity to methyl prednisolone affects cadaver kidney graft survival. *Lancet* 2: 1296–1297

113 Werner S, Thoren M, Gusafasson JA, Bronnegard M (1992) Glucocorticoid receptor abnormalities in fibroblasts from patients with idiopathis resistance of dexamethasone diagnosed when evaluated for adrenocortical disorders. *J Clin Endocrinol Metab* 75: 1005–1009

114 Moalli P, Rosen S (1994) Glucocorticoid receptors and resistance to glucocorticoids in hematologic malignancies. *Leukemia Lymphoma* 15: 363–374

115 Ray DW, Littlewood AC, Clark AJL, Davis JRE, White A (1994) Human small cell lung cancer cell lines expressing the propiomelanocortin gene have aberrant glucocorticoid receptor function. *J Clin Invest* 93: 1625–1630

116 Chikanza IC, Panayi GS (1993) The effects of hydrocortisone on *in vitro* lymphocytes proliferation and interleukin-2 and –4 production in corticosteroid sensitive and resistant subjects. *Eur J Clin Invest* 23: 845–850

117 Sher ER, Leung DYM, Surs W, Kam JC, Zieg G, Kamada AK, Szefler SJ (1994) Steroid-resistant asthma. Cellular mechanisms contributing to inadequate response to glucocorticoid therapy. *J Clin Invest* 93: 33–39

118 Bamberger CM, Bamberger AM, de Castro Margaret Chrousos GP (1995) Glucocorticoid receptor *B*, a potential endogenous inhibitor of glucocorticoid action in humans. *J Clin Invest* 95: 2435–2441

119 Norbiato G, Bevilacqua M, Vago T (1992) Cortisol resistance in acquired immunodeficiency syndrome. *J Clin Endocrinol Metab* 74: 608–613

120 Leung DYM, Hamid Q, Vottero A, Szefler SJ, Surs W, Minshall E, Chrousos GP, Klemm DJ (1997) Association of glucocorticoid insensitivity with increased expression of glucocorticoid receptor beta. *J Exp Med* 186: 1567–1574

121 Adcock IM, Lane SJ, Brown CR, Peters MJ, Lee TH, Barnes PJ (1995) Differences in binding of glucocorticoid receptor to DNA in steroid-resistant asthma. *J Immunol* 154: 3500–3505

122 Almawi WY, Lipman ML, Stevens AC, Zanker B, Hadro ET, Strom TB (1991) Abrogation of glucocorticoid mediated inhibition of T cell proliferation by the synergistic action of IL-1, IL-6 and IFN-gamma. *J Immunol* 146: 3523–3537

123 Kam JC, Szefler SJ, Surs W, Sher ER, Leung DYM (1993) Combination IL-2 and IL-4 reduced glucocorticoid receptor-binding affinity and T cell response to glucocorticoids[1]. *J Immunol* 151: 3460

124 Braack A, Tieener HL, Younge BR, Kaltschmidt C, Weyand CM, Goronzy (1997) Glucocorticoid-mediated repression of cytokine gene transcription in human arteritis-SCID chimeras. *J Clin Invest* 99: 28442–28450

125 Vayssiere BM, Dupont S, Choquart A, Petit F, Garcia T, Marchandeau C, Gronemeyer H, Resche-Rigon M (1997) Synthetic glucocorticoids that dissociate transactivation and AP-1 transrepression exhibit antiinflammatory activity *in vivo*. *Mol Endocrinol* 11: 1245–1255

Current perspectives in glucocorticoid biology

Glucocorticoids
ed. by N.J. Goulding and R.J. Flower
© 2001 Birkhäuser Verlag/Switzerland

Glucocorticoids and leukocyte adhesion

Costantino Pitzalis[1], Niccoló Pipitone[1] and Mauro Perretti [2]

[1] *Rheumatology Unit, GKT School of Medicine, Guy's Campus, London SE1 9RT, UK*
[2] *Department of Biochemical Pharmacology, The William Harvey Research Institute, Charterhouse Square, London EC1M 6BQ, UK*

Introduction

Adrenal glucocorticoids (GC) and their synthetic analogues are steroid molecules endowed with powerful anti-inflammatory and immunosuppressive properties. The mode of action of GC is very complex and not yet fully elucidated, but a number of mechanisms have been described. Traditionally, selected anti-inflammatory actions of GC have been largely ascribed to the synthesis of a protein termed lipocortin 1 or annexin 1 (AnxA1), which inhibits phospholipase A_2 activity with subsequent reduction in arachidonic acid release from the cell membrane and pro-inflammatory eicosanoid production [1, 2]. The immunosuppressive effect, on the other hand, is thought to be related to the inhibition of several immune functions, such as cytotoxicity, phagocytosis, and the synthesis of inflammatory cytokines like TNF-α, IL-1, IL-2 and IL-8 [3].

More recently, it has been realized that an additional important mechanism by which GC exert their effect is related to their GC capacity to interfere with intercellular adhesion processes. These are instrumental in mediating the adhesion of circulating leukocytes to vascular endothelial cells and their extravasation into peripheral tissues, where they form the cellular infiltrate typical of inflammatory lesions. Within the inflamed tissues, adhesion processes facilitate homotypic and heterotypic intercellular interactions that are essential for antigen presentation and cell activation. In addition, the adhesion of these cells to extracellular matrix allows the retention of blood-borne cells at sites of inflammation [4]. GC have the potential to interfere with virtually each of these processes by multiple mechanisms, and this capacity is being increasingly recognized as central to their anti-inflammatory and immunosuppressive properties.

General mechanisms of leukocyte migration

One of the earliest events in inflammation is leukocyte extravasation. The process of leukocyte extravasation is fairly well characterized and can be

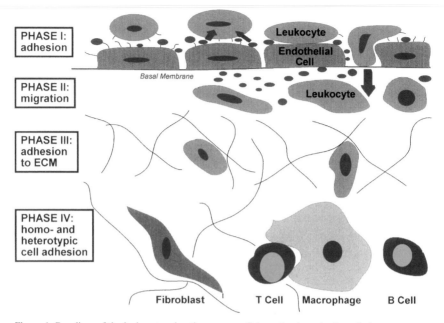

Figure 1. Paradigm of the leukocyte migration process. Schematized are the four distinct steps regulating leukocyte migration into inflamed tissues. See text for details and the adhesion molecules potentially involved in each distinct phase.

schematically divided into four sequential phases, each mediated by distinct classes of cell adhesion molecules (CAM) (Fig. 1) (the so-called "multistep model") [5, 6]. The *first step* (transient or intermittent adhesion) in this sequence is represented by leukocyte margination, which consists of leukocytes leaving the central stream of flowing blood cells in postcapillary venules, slowing down and starting rolling along the vessel wall. The molecules that mediate this step belong mainly to the selectins, a family of glycoproteins which includes L-selectin, E-selectin and P-selectin. L-selectin is principally expressed by leukocytes, while E- and P-selectin are expressed by EC and platelets. Selectins bind in an activation-independent fashion to oligosaccharidic receptors containing sialic acid residues [7]. This interaction between leukocytes and the endothelium of post-capillary venules is not very strong, however, it is sufficient to facilitate multiple transient contacts which provide the basis for the phenomenon of rolling. Usually, most rolling cells disengage and resume physiological flow, but during the course of an inflammatory reaction the number of cells that come to a halt increase dramatically [8]. The arrest of leukocytes onto the endothelial surface is largely mediated by leukocyte integrins, particularly $\beta 1$ (VLA-4) and $\beta 2$ (LFA-1 and MAC-1), and their respective endothelial counterparts, CAM-1, ICAM-1 and ICAM-2, which belong to the immunoglobulin super-family [9–12]. Integrins are normally expressed in a low-avidity, non-functional state in order to prevent random adhesion in the circulation, but can be triggered/activated (*second step*, cell activation) by inflammatory mediators such as bacterial wall components, complement products and, most importantly, chemoattractant cytokines (chemokines) [13, 14]. Chemokines mediate their effects by binding specific receptors characterised by a domain structure which spans the cell membrane seven times and signals through heterotrimeric GTP-binding proteins. Once activated, integrins are able to mediate adhesion of leukocytes to EC (*third step*, firm adhesion) by forming strong bonds with their endothelial counter-receptors. This enables leukocytes to stop and begin the process of trans-endothelial migration, resulting ultimately in cell extravasation into the inflamed tissues. Finally, the *fourth step* (diapedesis or emigration) involves the squeezing of leukocytes between EC and crossing of the basal membrane. Although we have limited understanding of the latter process, activated integrins probably play an important role as they appear to connect the external substratum with the intracellular cytoskeleton. PECAM-1 (CD31) expressed at the endothelial cell junctions is also involved in this specific step of the leukocyte extravasation process (Fig. 1).

Following extravasation, leukocytes localize to peripheral tissues, mainly in response to gradients of specific chemoattractants. The process of retention and accumulation of inflammatory cells within inflamed tissues is essentially mediated by the interactions that take place between leukocytes and components of the extracellular matrix (ECM) as well as by cell-cell adhesion phenomena. The interactions between cells and ECM are related to the expression of leukocyte integrins (mainly $\beta1$ integrins such as VLA-4 and VLA-5) that are able to bind to ECM constituents such as fibronectin, collagen and glycosaminoglycans [15, 16]. In this regard, the conspicuous absence of neutrophils from chronic inflammatory lesions at tissue level can be explained by the fact that neutrophils do not express $\beta1$ integrins. Intercellular adhesion processes are also largely mediated by integrins. In addition, lymphocytes can also bind LFA-3 positive cells *via* CD2, a member of the superfamily of immunoglobulins [9]. Again, given the virtually ubiquitous expression of LFA-3, this interaction can significantly contribute to bring lymphocytes in contact with several cell types.

Most of the CAM mentioned above undergo a significant up-regulation during inflammatory reactions, which, in turn, facilitates cell aggregation and the persistence of inflammation. CAM can induce and maintain cell activation in a two-fold manner. First, by anchoring cells to each other they make possible a whole array of processes that require close cell-cell contact, such as antigen presentation and cytotoxicity. Second, they can deliver stimulatory signals to the cells that result in cell activation (hence the name "co-stimulatory molecules" as in the case of the process of lymphocyte activation) [17, 18]. Therefore, CAM mediated events strongly contribute to the generation and perpetuation of chronic inflammatory infiltrates.

The effects of glucocorticoids on leukocyte adhesion mechanisms

Cronstein and colleagues first published GC ability to modulate the expression of CAM on human umbilical vein endothelial cells. Dexamethasone and cortisol were able to prevent up-regulation of E-selectin (CD62E) and ICAM-1 (CD54) on human endothelial cells following stimulation with lipolysaccharide (LPS) [19]. This observation initially generated some confusion since it was not confirmed by other laboratories [20]. Using an endothelial cell line (EA.hy926 cells, an hybridoma between HUVEC and the epithelioma A549 cells), again contrasting data were obtained: cell incubation with 1 μM dexamethasone reduced TNF-α and IL-1β-stimulated ICAM-1 up-regulation (an effect which was linked to a reduced neutrophil trans-endothelial migration) [21]. The synthetic GC suppressed LPS induced ICAM-1 induction, but not the up-regulation produced by the combination between TNF-α and INF-γ [22]. Addition of the latter cytokine overcomes the inhibition produced by the steroid as seen following co-incubation with LPS. However, GC ability to down-regulate endothelial expression of CAM is now an accepted mechanism of action for these potent anti-inflammatory drugs. Interference with the intracellular action of specific nuclear factors (e.g., NF-κB, see chapter by Paliogianni and Boumpas) is at the basis of GC inhibitory effect upon ICAM-1 [23, 24] and E-selectin [25] expression. Clinical data confirm the GC effect on CAM expression. For instance, topical application of mometasone reduces ICAM-1 expression in the psoriatic skin [26].

GC effects on endothelial cell adhesion molecules have been discussed in recent comprehensive reviews [27, 28]. Here, we will mainly focus on the modulatory action displayed by GC on leukocyte adhesion events.

Effects of GC on lymphocyte adhesion mechanisms

The concept that GC can interfere with lymphocyte binding to EC, the first step in the process of lymphocyte migration from the circulation into inflamed tissues, has been around since the early 1990s [29]. As stated above, studies focused mainly on the action of GC on the endothelium, rather than on the lymphocyte itself. Convincing evidence that GC could directly affect lymphocyte CAM expression was provided by subsequent *in vitro* work that showed that 24-h incubation of activated human lymphocytes with GC (dexamethasone 10^{-6} M) inhibited lymphocyte adhesion to a human endothelial cell line by approximately 35% [30]. In a similar way, GC were demonstrated to inhibit intercellular aggregation of activated lymphocytes by an average of 75% [30]. The inhibition of lymphocyte adhesion events appeared to be largely mediated by the down-regulation of the adhesion molecules LFA-1 and CD2, since there was a close correlation between cell aggregate formation and LFA-1/CD2 expression [30]. All these effects could be completely reversed using the GC receptor antagonist mifepristone (also known as RU 486).

Furthermore, GC treatment decreased the steady state mRNA levels of both LFA-1 and CD2 [30]. This suggested that GC could inhibit CAM gene transcription and/or decreas mRNA stability. Consistent with this hypothesis, a glucocorticoid response element (GRE) has been described upstream of the LFA-1 promoter [31]. By contrast, the effect of GC on CD2 mRNA steady state levels was less marked, and no GRE has been associated with the CD2 promoter, pointing to a different inhibitory mechanism for this molecule [30]. The inhibitory action of GC on LFA-1 expression was subsequently confirmed *in vivo* in a cohort of multiple sclerosis patients treated with oral and pulse GC, whereas CD2 expression inhibition in the same patients group was both less marked and less consistent [32]. The different magnitude of GC inhibition on different lymphocyte CAM is further underscored by the fact that GC were shown not to affect the expression of the $\beta1$ integrin VLA-4 on activated lymphocytes [33]. Again, this implies that lymphocyte CAM expression is regulated separately for each single molecule.

Many immunosuppressive and anti-inflammatory effects of GC are mediated by cytokines. On several cell types, pro-inflammatory cytokines such as TNF-α, IL-1β and IL-4 have been demonstrated to up-regulate adhesion molecule expression [34–38]. Thus, it is plausible that GC could down-regulate the expression of adhesion molecules, *inter alia*, through the inhibition of cytokine synthesis. In an *in vitro* model, TNF-α, IL-1, IL-4 and IL-10 were unable to affect adhesion molecule expression on resting human lymphocytes, however, IL-2 could up-regulate both LFA-1 and CD2 expression [39]. Similarly, IL-2, but not any of the other cytokines mentioned above, was able to reverse the inhibitory effect of GC on the up-regulation of LFA-1 and CD2 induced by TcR ligation [39]. These effects were paralleled by the capacity of IL-2 to reverse the inhibitory effect of GC on cell aggregate formation [39]. Therefore, this data supports the notion that GC can inhibit lymphocyte adhesion molecule expression also *via* an impairment of IL-2 secretion. This inhibitory effect is probably related to the capacity of GC to interfere with the activation of NF-κB and other transcription factors [40] that are necessary for the IL-2 promoter activation [41]. In contrast, GC do not affect the transcription rate of the IL-2R gene and may in fact induce IL-2R gene expression either directly or in synergy with IL-2 [42, 43]. The GC failure to repress the IL-2R gene is critically important as the unaltered expression of this receptor would make lymphocytes responsive to any IL-2 which can be produced by cells, thus escaping GC inhibition. This is a possible explanation for the common clinical observation that alternate day is less effective than daily GC therapy.

Effects of GC on neutrophil adhesion mechanisms

In the 1950s the first report on the clinical efficacy of cortisone in several rheumatic pathologies was published [44]. Since then experimental data have confirmed the anti-inflammatory profile displayed by GC and investigated the mechanisms responsible for their efficacy. The group of Susumu Tsurufuji has been among the first to investigate the potent anti-migratory action of dexamethasone in models of experimental inflammation [45, 46], and they studied how this effect was mediated by an interaction with the glucocorticoid receptor [47]. The high susceptibility of the process of leukocyte extravasation to GC has also been demonstrated in clinical settings. Single pulse methylprednisolone significantly reduced the number of neutrophils recovered from the synovial fluid of rheumatoid arthritis patients [48]. It is now clear that doses as low as 0.03 mg/kg of the potent synthetic GC dexamethasone [49] are able to potently inhibit the process of leukocyte recruitment in the rat.

As described above, the events which regulate the initial phases of leukocyte migration, i.e., the interaction with the endothelium of post-capillary venules, have been recently elucidated using techniques of intravital microscopy [28, 50]. A first study by Oda and Katori with the hamster cheek pouch microcirculation reported that dexamethasone was unable to modify any step of the leukocyte extravasation process when this was promoted by superfusion of the microvascular bed with formylated peptides [51]. However, a "retarding" effect of the GC on leukocyte movement into the sub-endothelial matrix was observed, leading to the proposition that GC might interfere with neutrophil passage through the basement membrane in the sub-endothelial space. In contrast, administration to hamsters of a dose of dexamethasone, able to inhibit cell recruitment into an inflamed cavity, reduced the extent of leukocyte emigration, but not rolling or adhesion, promoted by formyl-Met-Leu-Phe or substance P superfusion on the cheek pouch microcirculation [52]. Using the rat mesenteric microcirculation we have also been able to dissect the effect of this steroid on the different steps of leukocyte extravasation. When the interaction between circulating leukocytes and the post-capillary endothelium is promoted by direct acting chemoattractants (formylated peptides mentioned above or platelet-activating factor), dexamethasone potently inhibited cell emigration (the actual process of diapedesis) without affecting the up-stream events of cell rolling and adhesion. By contrast, when an endothelial activator such as interleukin-1 is used to promote the inflammatory reaction in a given microvascular bed, then the steroid is able to down-regulate the extent of cell adhesion as well as that of trans-endothelial passage [49]. On this basis, an additional GC effect on cell rolling upon application of non-specific stimuli (e.g., endotoxin or zymosan) was also proposed [53]. This hypothesis was confirmed by a study of Davenpeck et al., in which a 2 h-supraperfusion with lipopolysaccharide was used to promote neutrophil interaction with the endothelium of the rat mesenteric microcirculation [54]. Dexamethasone, used at a dose of 0.5 mg/kg which did not affect interleukin-1β-induced cell rolling [49], abrogated the rolling response to endotoxin.

Further evidence for a tonic control exerted by GC on the various steps of the leukocyte extravasation process are demonstrated in adrenalectomized rats [55]. All three migratory steps, promoted by the irritant carrageenin in the mesenteric vascular bed, are augmented following removal of endogenous GC by adrenalectomy, and suppressed by GC replenishment. These effects are mediated by the glucocorticoid receptor [55]. At this stage, it can therefore be concluded that GC are potent inhibitors of the process of leukocyte extravasation from the blood vessel into the interstitial tissue. The steps specifically affected by the GC depend upon several factors, including the GC dose, the administration regimen and the stimulus used to produce the inflammatory reaction. This clearly implicates that more than one molecular mechanism of action is operating in mediating GC effects on leukocyte adhesion and migration.

For example, GC are unable to affect neutrophil adhesion to endothelial monolayers *in vitro* [56], however an inhibitory effect is clearly measured under flow conditions as shown by the capacity of methylprednisolone to inhibit the adhesion of neutrophil flowing over IL-1β-activated endothelial monolayers [57]. Today, there is little doubt, even when direct-acting chemoattractants are used to elicit the inflammatory response, regarding the GC ability to modulate the neutrophil trafficking *in vivo*. Not many studies, however, have determined the potential GC effect on neutrophil adhesion molecule expression.

A single GC administration reduces CD18 expression on bovine neutrophils [58]. With respect to β2-integrin subtypes, expression of CD11b/CD18 is insensitive to single and repeated GC administration as seen in rat neutrophils either in basal conditions [59] or upon stimulation with LPS [60]. This differs from human neutrophils, which respond to GC treatment with reduction in CD11b and L-selectin levels [61, 62]. In man, up-regulation of neutrophil CD11b measured after anaesthesia is blunted by GC [63]. Studies in the rat have confirmed the latter effects, with dexamethasone preventing L-selectin shedding and CD11b/c integrin up-regulation in circulating neutrophils produced by LPS following perfusion of the rat mesentery [54]. Therefore, it would appear that similar to the situation described for lymphocytes, a distinction can be made between a *direct* GC effect on a specific neutrophil CAMs and *indirect* actions related to the modulation of leukocyte activation.

A recent study in the rabbit has functionally linked GC-induced granulocytosis to a bone marrow release of neutrophils bearing lower expression of L-selectin. Dexamethasone produced L-selectin shedding in the bone marrow itself [62]. It is unclear if this mechanism is a cause or a consequence of GC-induced granulocytosis, i.e., is L-selectin shedding a prerequisite to mobilise neutrophils from the marrow into the blood circulation? Similarly, how GC produce rapid shedding of this adhesion molecule, a phenomenon often associated to cell activation, remains at the moment obscure. It will be interesting to test the hypothesis that non-genomic GC actions (see below) might modulate cell release from the bone marrow.

Effects of GC on eosinophil adhesion mechanisms

Incubation of human eosinophils with dexamethasone for 24 h reduces CD11b up-regulation produced by PAF or eotaxin following *in vitro* activation [64].

This effect is the result of a reduction in basal CD11b levels. In the same culturing conditions, no effect on VLA-4 was detected. In mouse eosinophils, dexamethasone and budesonide, but not progesterone or testosterone, produce reduce basal CD11b expression in a concentration-dependent manner. This effect was prevented by addition of the GC receptor antagonist RU 486 [65]. The functional relevance of this finding is a lower degree of eosinophil migration in an *in vitro* chemotactic assay. Human eosinophil incubation with GC and interleukin-3 also produces down-regulation of CD11b levels [66]. Finally, administration of anti-inflammatory doses of dexamethasone to interleukin-5 transgenic mice also reduces CD11b expression on circulating eosinophils: the effect is dose- and time-dependent [65]. In view of the widespread application of GC in chronic allergic pathologies sustained by eosinophil accumulation, it is likely that GC ability to reduce integrin expression of this cell type may contribute to the clinical efficacy. Future studies in human volunteers and in asthmatic patients will test this hypothesis.

Effects of GC on monocyte adhesion mechanisms

Basal monocyte ICAM-1 levels are lowered following rat treatment with repeated doses of dexamethasone [59]. This effect is also measured on fully differentiated cells as peritoneal macrophages. Activation of the monocytic cell line, U937 cells, with IL-1β increases ICAM-1 levels, and this effect is again inhibited by GC. Similar inhibition of ICAM-1 up-regulation can also be seen on IL-1β-stimulated mouse macrophages [67]. De-activation of NF-κB briefly mentioned above is at the basis of GC effect upon ICAM-1 expression also in cells of the mono-myelocytic lineage [68].

Annexin 1 as mediator of the anti-migratory effect of dexamethasone

The 37 kDa protein annexin 1 (previously referred to as lipocortin 1) has long been proposed to mediate at least some of GC anti-inflammatory effects. After its discovery, annexin 1 biological actions were explained through an inhibition of the activity of the key pro-inflammatory enzyme phospholipase A_2, although other mechanisms of action are also possible [69–71].

With respect to the effects of GC on leukocyte recruitment, we observed that administration of dexamethasone to hamsters greatly promoted the "detachment" of leukocyte adherent to the cheek pouch microvessels [52]. This effect was seen irrespective of the stimulus applied and was abrogated by passive immunisation of hamsters against annexin 1. The efficacy of the polyclonal serum indicated that the antigen was some-how met in the microcirculation and/or in the inflamed tissue. More recently we have been able to see that most of annexin 1 contained in the cytoplasm of human neutrophils is externalised upon cell adhesion to endothelial monolayers [72]. This phenomenon results from a process of exocytosis of annexin 1 contained in the gelatinase granules, as demonstrated by electron microscopy [73], and by the fact that these sub-cellular organelles are mobilised selectively upon neutrophil adhesion [74]. The externalised protein can mimic the effects of dexamethasone in that it induces detachment of neutrophils adherent to mouse mesenteric post-capillary venules, for example following i.v. challenge with annexin 1 and annexin 1 peptide mimetics (N-terminus peptides) [75]. The molecular mechanism by which annexin 1 alters the fate of adherent cells is yet unknown, however it is clear that *the entire annexin 1 system is up-regulated following neutrophil adhesion to the endothelium*. In fact, not only the endogenous protein is secreted but its putative receptor is also up-regulated [76]. Future studies will determine the nature of the specific annexin 1 binding protein [77], and will also address the functional role that this GC-inducible protein may play in the process of recruitment of monocytes and lymphocytes. In an initial study, a different degree of protein mobilisation was seen upon cell adhesion among neutrophils, monocytes and lymphocytes prepared from the same volunteer [78].

Conclusions

It is increasingly clear that the mechanisms by which GC interfere with adhesion molecule expression are very complex. First, GC can act on different genes as well as transcription factors simultaneously. Second, adhesion molecule themselves are regulated differently depending on the cell types and the stimuli considered. For instance, TNF-α and IL-1 can upregulate CAM expression on endothelial cells and fibroblasts [79, 80], whereas lymphocyte CAM are upregulated by IL-2, but not TNF-α or IL-1. Third, GC may regulate CAM expression in response to different cytokines in different ways. To mention an example, GC were shown to inhibit endothelial E-selectin and ICAM-1 expression in response to LPS [19]. However, GC were able to prevent accumulation of E-selectin mRNA in response to LPS and IL-1β but not TNF-α, suggesting that different mechanisms are probably operating even within the same cell type in response to different stimuli [19]. Fourth, the expression of different adhesion molecule in response to the same stimulus may be more or less sensitive to the effect of GC. In this regard, we have already mentioned that the expression of the LFA-1 gene in response to TcR ligation is much more sensitive than the CD2 gene to the effects of GC both at the mRNA and the protein level. Finally, there are important differences in the responses of different individuals to the inhibitory action of GC on CAM expression, which may account, at least in part, for the various degrees of GC sensitivity observed in clinical practice.

The multiple mechanisms underlying the GC induced inhibition of CAM gene expression described above are often referred to as "genomic mechanisms" because they relate to the interference of GC with the transcriptional and post-transcriptional machinery involved in protein synthesis. Genomic mechanisms are widely considered responsible for the majority of effects displayed by GC. However, recently, there has been a renewed interest in those mechanisms that act independently of gene regulation (non-genomic mechanisms). The *non-genomic mechanisms* of GC have been less extensively investigated but their importance is increasingly recognised. They are characterised by a very rapid response (seconds/minutes) and by their insensitivity to inhibitors of gene transcription and protein synthesis such as actinomycin D and cycloheximide [81]. Such non-genomic effects could be mediated by a membrane receptor or be due to direct physicochemical interactions with cell membrane constituents including ion channels and membrane associated proteins. Irrespective of whether GC act *via* specific membrane receptors or *via* direct physicochemical mechanisms, GC binding to the cell membrane increases plasma membrane stability with profound effects on cell activation/response including modulation of phospholipid hydrolysis, generation of second messengers (e.g IP3), cation cycling and free radical production [81]. In addition, the mobilization of annexin 1 is also independent from genomic regulation.

Preliminary data suggests that non-genomic mechanisms may be of relevance to the action of GC on CAM function. *In vitro*, GC can inhibit the intercellular aggregation of lymphocytes induced by PMA within minutes (personal observation). Given the rapidity of this action, it is clear that non-genomic mechanisms must be operative. Similarly, GC can significantly inhibit the PMA induced expression of the LFA-1 activation epitope recognized by the mAb 24 on lymphocytes in as little as half an hour (personal observation). Therefore, it is likely that GC modulate adhesion mechanisms by regulating CAM activation and consequently their avidity/affinity status. Even more important, these mechanisms appear to have an *in vivo* correlate, since intravenous methylprednisolone pulse therapy inhibits neutrophil migration into rheumatoid joints very rapidly [82].

In conclusion, there is now compelling evidence that GC can affect directly leukocyte CAM expression, and that this action can account for at least part of the anti-inflammatory properties of GC. The mechanisms responsible are still incompletely defined, but they can certainly occur at multiple levels and may involve both genomic and non-genomic pathways. As novel, "dissociated" steroids with less metabolic side-effects are being actively developed [83], dissection of the mechanisms underlying modulation of CAM expression/function may offer new insights into the mode of action of GC. This may facilitate the creation of new agents with more selective anti-inflammatory properties.

References

1 Flower RJ (1990) Lipocortin. *Prog Clin Biol Res* 349: 11–25
2 Goulding NJ, Godolphin JL, Sharland PR, Peers SH, Sampson M, Maddison PJ, Flower RJ (1990) Anti-inflammatory lipocortin 1 production by peripheral blood leucocytes in response to hydrocortisone. *Lancet* 335(8703): 1416–1418

3 Boumpas DT, Paliogianni F, Anastassiou ED, Balow JE (1991) Glucocorticosteroid action on the immune system: molecular and cellular aspects. *Clin Exp Rheumatol* 9(4): 413–423
4 Pitzalis C (1996) The Michael Mason Prize Essay Role of adhesion mechanisms in the pathogenesis of chronic synovitis. *Brit J Rheumatol* 35(12): 1198–1215
5 Butcher EC (1992) Leukocyte-endothelial cell adhesion as an active, multi-step process: a combinatorial mechanism for specificity and diversity in leukocyte targeting. *Adv Exp Med Biol* 323: 181–194
6 Butcher EC (1991) Leukocyte-endothelial cell recognition: three (or more) steps to specificity and diversity. *Cell* 67(6): 1033–1036
7 Bevilacqua MP, Nelson RM (1993) Selectins. *J Clin Invest* 91(2): 379–387
8 Atherton A, Born GV (1972) Quantitative investigations of the adhesiveness of circulating polymorphonuclear leucocytes to blood vessel walls. *J Physiol* 222(2): 447–474
9 Springer TA (1990) Adhesion receptors of the immune system. *Nature* 346(6283): 425–434
10 Kornberg L, Earp HS, Parsons JT, Schaller M, Juliano RL (1992) Cell adhesion or integrin clustering increases phosphorylation of a focal adhesion-associated tyrosine kinase. *J Biol Chem* 267(33): 23439–23442
11 Hogg N, Landis RC (1993) Adhesion molecules in cell interactions. *Curr Opin Immunol* 5(3): 383–390
12 Hogg N, Harvey J, Cabanas C, Landis RC (1993) Control of leukocyte integrin activation. *Amer Rev Respir Dis* 148(6 Pt 2): S55–S59
13 Schall TJ, Bacon KB (1994) Chemokines, leukocyte trafficking, and inflammation. *Curr Opin Immunol* 6(6): 865–873
14 Baggiolini M, Dewald B, Moser B (1997) Human chemokines: an update. *Annu Rev Immunol* 15: 675–705
15 Hemler ME (1988) Adhesive protein receptors on hematopoietic cells. *Immunol Today* 9(4): 109–113
16 Rodriguez RM, Pitzalis C, Kingsley GH, Henderson E, Humphries MJ, Panayi GS (1992) T lymphocyte adhesion to fibronectin (FN): a possible mechanism for T cell accumulation in the rheumatoid joint. *Clin Exp Immunol* 89(3): 439–445
17 Van Seventer GA, Shimizu Y, Horgan KJ, Shaw S (1990) The LFA-1 ligand ICAM-1 provides an important costimulatory signal for T cell receptor-mediated activation of resting T cells. *J Immunol* 144(12): 4579–4586
18 Van Seventer GA, Newman W, Shimizu Y, Nutman TB, Tanaka Y, Horgan KJ, Gopal TV, Ennis E, O'Sullivan D, Grey H et al (1991) Analysis of T cell stimulation by superantigen plus major histocompatibility complex class II molecules or by CD3 monoclonal antibody: costimulation by purified adhesion ligands VCAM-1, ICAM-1, but not ELAM-1. *J Exp Med* 174(4): 901–913
19 Cronstein BN, Kimmel SC, Levin RI, Martiniuk F, Weissmann G (1992) A mechanism for the antiinflammatory effects of corticosteroids: the glucocorticoid receptor regulates leukocyte adhesion to endothelial cells and expression of endothelial-leukocyte adhesion molecule 1 and intercellular adhesion molecule 1. *Proc Natl Acad Sci USA* 89(21): 9991–9995
20 Fosyth KD, Talbot V (1992) Role of glucocorticoids in neutrophil and endothelial adhesion molecule expression and function. *Med Inflamm* 1: 101–106
21 Wheller SK, Perretti M (1997) Dexamethasone inhibits cytokine-induced intercellular adhesion molecule-1 up-regulation on endothelial cell lines. *Eur J Pharmacol* 331(1): 65–71
22 Burke-Gaffney A, Hellewell PG (1996) Regulation of ICAM-1 by dexamethasone in a human vascular endothelial cell line EAhy926. *Amer J Physiol* 270(2 Pt 1):C552–C561
23 Caldenhoven E, Liden J, Wissink S, Van de Stolpe A, Raaijmakers J, Koenderman L, Okret S, Gustafsson JA, van der Saag PT (1995) Negative cross-talk between RelA and the glucocorticoid receptor: a possible mechanism for the antiinflammatory action of glucocorticoids. *Mol Endocrinol* 9(4): 401–412
24 Van de Stolpe A, Caldenhoven E, Stade BG, Koenderman L, Raaijmakers JA, Johnson JP, van der Saag PT (1994) 12-O-tetradecanoylphorbol-13-acetate- and tumor necrosis factor alpha-mediated induction of intercellular adhesion molecule-1 is inhibited by dexamethasone. Functional analysis of the human intercellular adhesion molecular-1 promoter. *J Biol Chem* 269(8): 6185–6192
25 Brostjan C, Anrather J, Csizmadia V, Natarajan G, Winkler H (1997) Glucocorticoids inhibit E-selectin expression by targeting NF-kappaB and not ATF/c-Jun. *J Immunol* 158(8): 3836–3844
26 Berti E, Cerri A, Marzano AV, Richelda R, Bianchi B, Caputo R (1998) Mometasone furoate decreases adhesion molecule expression in psoriasis. *Eur J Dermatol* 8(6): 421–426

27 Henricks PA, Nijkamp FP (1998) Pharmacological modulation of cell adhesion molecules. *Eur J Pharmacol* 344(1): 1–13

28 Panes J, Perry M, Granger DN (1999) Leukocyte-endothelial cell adhesion: avenues for therapeutic intervention. *Brit J Pharmacol* 126(3): 537–550

29 Eguchi K, Kawakami A, Nakashima M, Ida H, Sakito S, Matsuoka N, Terada K, Sakai M, Kawabe Y, Fukuda T et al (1992) Interferon-alpha and dexamethasone inhibit adhesion of T cells to endothelial cells and synovial cells. *Clin Exp Immunol* 88(3): 448–454

30 Pitzalis C, Pipitone N, Bajocchi G, Hall M, Goulding N, Lee A, Kingsley G, Lanchbury J, Panayi G (1997) Corticosteroids inhibit lymphocyte binding to endothelium and intercellular adhesion: an additional mechanism for their anti-inflammatory and immunosuppressive effect. *J Immunol* 158(10): 5007–5016

31 Nueda A, Lopez-Cabrera M, Vara A, Corbi AL (1993) Characterization of the CD11a (alpha L, LFA-1 alpha) integrin gene promoter. *J Biol Chem* 268(26): 19305–19311

32 Pitzalis C, Sharrack B, Gray IA, Lee A, Hughes RA (1997) Comparison of the effects of oral *versus* intravenous methylprednisolone regimens on peripheral blood T lymphocyte adhesion molecule expression, T cell subsets distribution and TNF alpha concentrations in multiple sclerosis. *J Neuroimmunol* 74(1–2): 62–68

33 Hughes JM, Sewell WA, Black JL, Armour CL (1996) Effect of dexamethasone on expression of adhesion molecules on CD4+ lymphocytes. *Amer J Physiol* 271(1 Pt 1): L79–84

34 Cicuttini FM, Martin M, Boyd AW (1994) Cytokine induction of adhesion molecules on synovial type B cells. *J Rheumatol* 21(3): 406–412

35 Gerritsen ME, Niedbala MJ, Szczepanski A, Carley WW (1993) Cytokine activation of human macro- and microvessel-derived endothelial cells. Blood Cells 19(2): 325–339; discussion 340–342

36 Satoh J, Kastrukoff LF, Kim SU (1991) Cytokine-induced expression of intercellular adhesion molecule-1 (ICAM-1) in cultured human oligodendrocytes and astrocytes. *J Neuropathol Exp Neurol* 50(3): 215–226

37 Doucet C, Brouty-Boye D, Pottin-Clemenceau C, Jasmin C, Canonica GW, Azzarone B (1998) IL-4 and IL-13 specifically increase adhesion molecule and inflammatory cytokine expression in human lung fibroblasts. *Int Immunol* 10(10): 1421–1433

38 Gundel R, Lindell D, Harris P, Fournel M, Jesmok G, Gerritsen ME (1996) IL-4 induced leucocyte trafficking in cynomolgus monkeys: correlation with expression of adhesion molecules and chemokine generation. *Clin Exp Allergy* 26(6): 719–729

39 Pipitone N, Goulding NJ, Marcolongo RF, Panayi GS, Pitzalis C (2000) The glucocorticoid induced LFA-1 and CD2 adhesion molecule inhibition is reversed by IL-2, but not other cytokines. (submitted)

40 Wissink S, van Heerde EC, vand der Burg B, van der Saag PT (1998) A dual mechanism mediates repression of NF-kappaB activity by glucocorticoids. *Mol Endocrinol* 12(3): 355–363

41 Hughes CC, Pober JS (1996) Transcriptional regulation of the interleukin-2 gene in normal human peripheral blood T cells. Convergence of costimulatory signals and differences from transformed T cells. *J Biol Chem* 271(10): 5369–5377

42 Boumpas DT, Anastassiou ED, Older SA, Tsokos GC, Nelson DL, Balow JE (1991) Dexamethasone inhibits human interleukin 2 but not interleukin 2 receptor gene expression *in vitro* at the level of nuclear transcription. *J Clin Invest* 87(5): 1739–1747

43 Lamas M, Sanz E, Martin-Parras L, Espel E, Sperisen P, Collins M, Silva AG (1993) Glucocorticoid hormones upregulate interleukin 2 receptor alpha gene expression. Cellular Immunology 151(2): 437–450

44 Hench PS, Kendall EC, Slocumb CH (1950) Effects of cortisone acetate and pituitary ACTH on rheumatoid arthritis, rheumatic fever and certain other conditions: a study of clinical physiology. *Arch Intern Med* 85: 545

45 Ishikawa H, Mori Y, Tsurufuji S (1969) The characteristic feature of glucocorticoids after local application with reference to leucocyte migration and protein exudation. *Eur J Pharmacol* 7(2): 201–205

46 Konno S, Tsurufuji S (1983) Induction of zymosan-air-pouch inflammation in rats and its characterization with reference to the effects of anticomplementary and anti-inflammatory agents. *Brit J Pharmacol* 80(2): 269–277

47 Tsurufuji S, Sugio K, Takemasa F (1979) The role of glucocorticoid receptor and gene expression in the anti-inflammatory action of dexamethasone. *Nature* 280(5721): 408–410

48 Youssef P, Roberts-Thomson P, Ahern M, Smith M (1995) Pulse methylprednisolone in rheumatoid arthritis: effects on peripheral blood and synovial fluid neutrophil surface phenotype. *J Rheumatol* 22(11): 2065–2071

49 Tailor A, Flower RJ, Perretti M (1997) Dexamethasone inhibits leukocyte emigration in rat mesenteric post-capillary venules: an intravital microscopy study. *J Leukocyte Biol* 62(3): 301–308

50 Granger DN, Kubes P (1994) The microcirculation and inflammation: modulation of leukocyte-endothelial cell adhesion. *J Leukocyte Biol* 55(5): 662–675

51 Oda T, Katori M (1992) Inhibition site of dexamethasone on extravasation of polymorphonuclear leukocytes in the hamster cheek pouch microcirculation. *J Leukocyte Biol* 52(3): 337–342

52 Mancuso F, Flower RJ, Perretti M (1995) Leukocyte transmigration, but not rolling or adhesion, is selectively inhibited by dexamethasone in the hamster post-capillary venule. Involvement of endogenous lipocortin 1. *J Immunol* 155(1): 377–386

53 Perretti M (1998) Lipocortin 1 and chemokine modulation of granulocyte and monocyte accumulation in experimental inflammation. *Gen Pharmacol* 31(4): 545–552

54 Davenpeck KL, Zagorski J, Schleimer RP, Bochner BS (1998) Lipopolysaccharide-induced leukocyte rolling and adhesion in the rat mesenteric microcirculation: regulation by glucocorticoids and role of cytokines. *J Immunol* 161(12): 6861–6870

55 Farsky SP, Sannomiya P, Garcia-Leme J (1995) Secreted glucocorticoids regulate leukocyte-endothelial interactions in inflammation. A direct vital microscopic study. *J Leukocyte Biol* 57(3): 379–386

56 Schleimer RP, Freeland HS, Peters SP, Brown KE, Derse CP (1989) An assessment of the effects of glucocorticoids on degranulation, chemotaxis, binding to vascular endothelium and formation of leukotriene B4 by purified human neutrophils. *J Pharmacol Exp Therapeut* 250(2): 598–605

57 Yoshida N, Yoshikawa T, Nakamura Y, Takenaka S, Sakamoto K, Manabe H, Nakagawa S, Kondo M (1997) Methylprednisolone inhibits neutrophil-endothelial cell interactions induced by interleukin-1beta under flow conditions. *Life Sci* 60(25): 2341–2347

58 Burton JL, Kehrli ME, Jr Kapil S, Horst RL (1995) Regulation of L-selectin and CD18 on bovine neutrophils by glucocorticoids: effects of cortisol and dexamethasone. *J Leukocyte Biol* 57(2): 317–325

59 Tailor A, Das AM, Getting SJ, Flower RJ, Perretti M (1997) Subacute treatment of rats with dexamethasone reduces ICAM-1 levels on circulating monocytes. *Biochem Biophys Res Commun* 231(3): 675–678

60 O'Leary EC, Marder P, Zuckerman SH (1996) Glucocorticoid effects in an endotoxin-induced rat pulmonary inflammation model: differential effects on neutrophil influx, integrin expression, and inflammatory mediators. *Amer J Respir Cell Mol Biol* 15(1): 97–106

61 Filep JG, Delalandre A, Payette Y, Foldes-Filep E (1997) Glucocorticoid receptor regulates expression of L-selectin and CD11/CD18 on human neutrophils [see comments]. *Circulation* 96(1): 295–301

62 Nakagawa M, Bondy GP, Waisman D, Minshall D, Hogg JC, van Eeden SF (1999) The effect of glucocorticoids on the expression of L-selectin on polymorphonuclear leukocyte. *Blood* 93(8): 2730–2737

63 Hill ME, Bird IN, Daniels RH, Elmore MA, Finnen MJ (1994) Endothelial cell-associated platelet-activating factor primes neutrophils for enhanced superoxide production and arachidonic acid release during adhesion to but not transmigration across IL-1 beta-treated endothelial monolayers. *J Immunol* 153(8): 3673–3683

64 DASAM, Lim LHK, Flower RJ, Perretti M (1997) Dexamethasone reduces cell surface levels of CD11b on human eosinophils. *Med Inflamm* 6: 363–367

65 Lim LHK, Flower RJ, Perretti M, Das AM (2000) Glucocorticoid receptor activation reduces CD11b and CD49d levels on murine eosinophils: characterization and functional relevance. *Amer J Resp Cell Mol Biol* 22: 693–701

66 Hartnell A, Kay AB, Wardlaw AJ (1992) Interleukin-3-induced up-regulation of CR3 expression on human eosinophils is inhibited by dexamethasone. *Immunology* 77(4): 488–493

67 Perretti M, Wheller SK, Harris JG, Flower RJ (1996) Modulation of ICAM-1 levels on U-937 cells and mouse macrophages by interleukin-1 beta and dexamethasone. *Biochem Biophys Res Commun* 223(1): 112–117

68 van der Saag PT, Caldenhoven E, Van de Stolpe A (1996) Molecular mechanisms of steroid action: a novel type of cross-talk between glucocorticoids and NF-kappa B transcription factors. *Eur Respir J (Suppl)* 22: 146s–53s

69 Flower RJ (1988) Eleventh Gaddum memorial lecture. Lipocortin and the mechanism of action of the glucocorticoids. *Brit J Pharmacol* 94(4): 987–1015

70 Ahluwalia A, Buckingham JC, Croxtall JD, Flower RJ, Goulding NJ, Peretti M (1996) The biology of annexin I. *In*: BA Seaton (ed.) *Annexins: molecular structure to cellular function*. R.G. Landes, Austin, 161–199

71 Kim KM, Kim DK, Park YM, Kim CK, Na DS (1994) Annexin-I inhibits phospholipase A2 by specific interaction, not by substrate depletion. *FEBS Lett* 343(3): 251–255

72 Perretti M, Croxtall JD, Wheller SK, Goulding NJ, Hannon R, Flower RJ (1996) Mobilizing lipocortin 1 in adherent human leukocytes downregulates their transmigration. *Nat Med* 2(11): 1259–1262

73 Perretti M, Christian H, Wheller SK, Aiello I, Mugridge KG, Morris JF, Flower RJ, Goulding NJ (2000) Annexin I is stored within gelatinase granules of human neutrophil and mobilised on the cell surface upon adhesion but not phagocytosis. *Cell Biol Int* 24: 163–174

74 Borregaard N, Cowland JB (1997) Granules of the human neutrophilic polymorphonuclear leukocyte. *Blood* 89(10): 3503–3521

75 Lim LH, Solito E, Russo-Marie F, Flower RJ, Perretti M (1998) Promoting detachment of neutrophils adherent to murine postcapillary venules to control inflammation: effect of lipocortin 1. *Proc Natl Acad Sci USA* 95(24): 14535–14539

76 Euzger E, Flower RJ, Goulding NJ, Perretti M (1999) Differential modulation of annexin I binding sites on monocytes and neutrophils. *Med Inflamm* 8: 53–62

77 Goulding NJ, Pan L, Wardwell K, Guyre VC, Guyre PM (1996) Evidence for specific annexin I-binding proteins on human monocytes. *Biochem J* 316(Pt 2): 593–597

78 Perretti M, Wheller SK, Flower RJ, Wahid S, Pitzalis C (1999) Modulation of cellular annexin I in human leukocytes infiltrating DTH skin reactions. *J Leukocyte Biol* 65(5): 583–589

79 Braun M, Pietsch P, Felix SB, Baumann G (1995) Modulation of intercellular adhesion molecule-1 and vascular cell adhesion molecule-1 on human coronary smooth muscle cells by cytokines. *J Mol Cell Cardiol* 27(12): 2571–2579

80 Krzesicki RF, Fleming WE, Winterrowd GE, Hatfield CA, Sanders ME, Chin JE (1991) T lymphocyte adhesion to human synovial fibroblasts. Role of cytokines and the interaction between intercellular adhesion molecule 1 and CD11a/CD18. *Arthritis Rheumatism* 34(10): 1245–1253

81 Buttgereit F, Wehling M, Burmester GR (1998) A new hypothesis of modular glucocorticoid actions: steroid treatment of rheumatic diseases revisited [comment]. *Arthritis Rheumatism* 41(5): 761–767

82 Youssef PP, Cormack J, Evill CA, Peter DT, Roberts-Thomson PJ, Ahern MJ, Smith MD (1996) Neutrophil trafficking into inflamed joints in patients with rheumatoid arthritis, and the effects of methylprednisolone [see comments]. *Arthritis Rheumatism* 39(2): 216–225

83 Barnes PJ (1998) Anti-inflammatory actions of glucocorticoids: molecular mechanisms [editorial]. *Clin Sci* 94(6): 557–572

Annexin I as a mediator of glucocorticoid action

Jamie D. Croxtall

Department of Biochemical Pharmacology, The William Harvey Institute, St. Bartholomew's and the Royal London School of Medicine & Dentistry (Queen Mary and Westfield College), Charterhouse Square, London EC1M 6BQ, UK

Since the 1950s glucocorticoids have been used extensively in the treatment of inflammatory diseases and despite several undesirable side-effects they still remain as one of the most important drugs to control inflammation. Little was known about the mechanism of action of glucocorticoids until the 1970s when a detailed study of their molecular actions was first began. Since that time our knowledge of the cellular mechanisms that mediate the effects of glucocorticoids has grown considerably. Briefly, following an interaction with specific intracellular receptors, and in concert with other transcription factors, the glucocorticoid receptor complex binds to specific DNA response elements within the promoter sequences of key target genes. As a result of this interaction the expression of many pro-inflammatory mediators is suppressed. However, it is now clear that this process also up-regulates the expression of other mediators that have potent anti-inflammatory properties. This chapter reviews the evidence of one such anti-inflammatory mediator of glucocorticoid action - annexin I.

The 1970s were an exciting period of discovery. During this time, cyclooxygenase (COX) was discovered as the enzyme which converted arachidonic acid (liberated from phospholipid membranes by phospholipase A_2) to pro-inflammatory prostaglandins (PGs) [1]. Furthermore, COX was found to be the site of action of aspirin and other non-steroidal anti-inflammatory drugs (NSAIDS) which, by inhibiting the catalytic activity of the enzyme, blocked the formation of PGs [2]. Glucocorticoids were also known to block the formation of PGs, but, in cell-free assays of COX preparations it was clear that the catalytic activity of the enzyme was unaffected. However, unlike aspirin and the NSAIDS, glucocorticoids were also known to block the release of arachidonic acid [3]. It therefore seemed likely that the site of action of glucocorticoids was by inhibition of PLA_2 activity. Again, using cell-free assays of PLA_2 preparations, the activity of the enzyme itself was unaffected by glucocorticoid treatment. However, in whole-cell systems the suppression of PLA_2 activity was reversed by inhibitors of protein synthesis [4]. In other words, the phospolipase-inhibitory effect of glucocorticoids requires the synthesis of mediator proteins. To this day, this has remained as a fundamental premise of the action of glucocorticoids.

Glucocorticoids inhibit PLA$_2$ activity *via* the induction of mediator proteins

The discovery of likely candidates for these mediators of glucocorticoid action occurred almost simultaneously in three different laboratories. Using inflammatory model systems of either activated neutrophils, renal medullary cells or peritoneal macrophages it was shown that the glucocorticoid inhibition of arachidonic acid release was dependent on the synthesis of mediatory proteins. More importantly, these groups were able to demonstrate that in each system, glucocorticoid treatment resulted in the production of a factor that mimicked the inhibitory action of the steroid itself. This factor was heat sensitive and destroyed by proteolytic activity. Early attempts at characterization of these factors were unclear but it subsequently became apparent that each group had in fact identified the same 37 kDa protein, which we now call annexin I [5–7].

It is perhaps now hard to re-create the excitement of that discovery, but the implications were immediately obvious to all involved. Principally, that by using annexin I as an anti-inflammatory agent one could selectively down-regulate PLA$_2$ activity and thus prostanoid release without incurring the deleterious side-effects associated with glucocorticoid therapy. There has since followed an intense period of investigation into the mechanism of induction and the cellular actions of annexin I.

Annexin I is a glucocorticoid inducible protein

Induction of annexin I by glucocorticoids has now been reported in many systems including human monocytes both *in vivo* and *in vitro*, rat macrophage and thymus *in vivo*, human bronchioalveolar lavage fluid, rat pituitary and also following topical application to human skin. Furthermore, adrenalectomy decreases annexin I expression *in vivo*. Despite this, a failure to demonstrate an induction in some systems has led some to doubt the validity of annexin I as a mediator of glucocorticoid action.

Perhaps the greatest insight into the nature of annexin I inducibility has come from several studies using *in vitro* cell culture systems from which it is now apparent that the mechanism is more complex than originally thought. Using an immature monocytic cell line (U937 cells) a poor response is seen to glucocorticoids without prior treatment with phorbol ester [8]. In other words, undifferentiated cells respond less well than differentiated cells. Furthermore, the differentiation procedure itself also elevates annexin I expression indicating that the protein is inducible by other mechanisms. Using the same cell system it is apparent that serum-derived cytokines are also capable of inducing annexin I. Similarly, human fibroblasts cultured in serum containing media express elevated levels of annexin I following a change of media – and this is mimicked by the addition of EGF.

For these reasons a simplified system of cell culture was developed using the A549 human lung adenocarcinoma cell line [9]. These cells are highly sensitive to glucocorticoids, grow in the absence of serum and do not require pre-differentiation to attain a responsive state. Glucocorticoids readily induce annexin I expression in A549 cells grown in defined media [9]. The glucocorticoid inhibition of PLA_2 activity and arachidonic acid release is reversed by the presence of neutralizing antibodies and anti-sense oligonucleotides to annexin I [10, 11]. Furthermore purified annexin I mimics the action of glucocorticoids in these cells. So in some respects, the A549 cell culture system provides a reliable *in vitro* model that in many ways resembles some aspects of the inflammatory models described above where annexin I was first observed. For example, glucocorticoid-induced annexin I is removed from the peritoneal cavity or from lung lavage by washing with a low calcium-containing buffer. So too is inducible annexin I removed from the monolayer of A549 cells by washing with PBS-EDTA. In fact, it is clear from further studies with these cells that the annexin I removed by this procedure represents the most significant inducible pool of the protein. The importance of the sub-cellular redistribution of annexin I following glucocorticoid treatment is something that has been repeatedly observed in several systems. Not only is newly synthesised annexin I released on the surface of U937 and A549 cells *in vitro*, but also in rat and human peritoneal leukocytes *in vivo*. Furthermore, this release of annexin I may occur very rapidly (i.e., within minutes) as shown most convincingly in the rat anterior pituitary where the short-term actions of glucocorticoids are clearly distinguished from longer term actions. This has led to some authors describing a rapid (protein synthesis-independent) and delayed (protein synthesis-dependent) effect of glucocorticoid induction of annexin I as two distinct events [12].

Taken together these observations are indicative of a rapid mobilization of annexin I to cell membranes (and perhaps followed by a longer term re-synthesis process) following glucocorticoid treatment. If the complicating effects of serum derived growth factors or differentiating agents are not taken into account then this process may well be obscured. More importantly, if treated cells are processed in low calcium buffers then this membrane bound pool of annexin I will be lost. This alone may account for many of the failures to report an induction of the protein.

Due to the pluripotent nature of glucocorticoids a great many cellular processes are affected by their action. Indeed, as much as 1% of the genome is believed to be under direct control of glucocorticoids. Therefore, a key question is how many of these effects are mediated *via* the induction of annexin I?

Annexin I mediated effects of glucocorticoids

The development of neutralizing anti-sera to annexin I (and more recently, anti-sense oligonucleotides) which block its biological actions has enabled experimental strategies to be developed which determine whether the protein is a mediator of glucocorticoid effects in a number of systems. Most significantly perhaps, are that a number of anti-inflammatory actions of glucocorticoids have been shown to be reversed in this manner. These include inhibition of cytokine induced fever and cell migration, carrageenin paw oedema and lipid mediator release. Furthermore, the physiological feedback mechanism of glucocorticoids on the anterior pituitary gland is also reversed by annexin I anti-serum. Also, significantly, the growth inhibitory and differentiating effects of glucocorticoids have been shown to be mediated by annexin I in several cell systems.

These observations were further supported with the development of a recombinant form of annexin I (and subsequently peptide fragments) which mimicked the activity of glucocorticoids in many of these models. For example, recombinant annexin I is effective in inhibiting paw oedema and neutrophil migration [13, 14]. Similarly, a truncated form of recombinant annexin I (approximately half the protein) is active in the anterior pituitary gland and also retains potent anti-pyretic activity [15, 16]. Furthermore, both these forms of annexin I (and smaller peptide fragments) effectively inhibit the generation of arachidonic acid and the release of PGE_2 from A549 cells, and thereby inhibit cell growth [17]. Taken together these observations provide convincing evidence that annexin I is a glucocorticoid-inducible protein that mediates many of the anti-inflammatory actions of the steroid. Furthermore, a purified source of the protein mimics these actions of glucocorticoids. This period was a very exciting one in the discovery of the actions of annexin I which appeared to vindicate the original premise of this mediator as an alternative pharmacological agent to glucocorticoids. However, this was not so clear cut as originally thought. Firstly, as elaborated at the beginning of this chapter, glucocorticoids inhibit the activity of PLA_2 *via* inducible mediator proteins. In the inflammatory models discussed above the inhibition of PLA_2 activity by glucocorticoids is central to their anti-inflammatory effect. Therefore, annexin I must have demonstrable PLA_2 inhibitory properties.

Is annexin I an inhibitor of PLA_2?

PLA_2 is the enzyme responsible for the catalysis of membrane phospholipid to release arachidonic acid which is then subsequently converted to a variety of eicosanoid metabolites. As such, arachidonic acid does not exist in free form, rather it is released as required by PLA_2 and immediately converted. This implies that PLA_2 is the rate limiting step in the generation of pro-inflammatory mediators. Clearly, the control of PLA_2 activity is central to regulating the inflammatory process. It was originally assumed that PLA_2 had only one form and the main source of this for experimental purposes was derived from porcine pancreas. This form of PLA_2 has a molecular weight of around 14 kDa, a requirement for mM concentrations of calcium for maximal catalytic activity and is relatively unselective in its ability to digest different forms of phospholipid. A very similar form of PLA_2 is found secreted by gastric mucosal cells and is thought to play an important physiological role in lipid digestion. More importantly perhaps, it is also found secreted in elevated amounts at inflammatory sites, and although it may play a beneficial role in pathogen destruction, it is also thought to contribute to the pathological process of tissue damage through its digestive properties. These secretory forms of PLA_2 (hereafter termed $sPLA_2$) were the original forms used in experiments to determine the inhibitory properties of annexin I. Extensive enzyme kinetic assays revealed that, at mM concentrations of calcium, annexin I was indeed an inhibitor of $sPLA_2$, but this appeared to be through a mechanism of substrate sequestration rather than by direct enzymatic inhibition [18]. This was of course hugely disappointing to those involved as it implied that the original premise of annexin I as a selective inhibitory mediator of glucocorticoid action was flawed. In retrospect, these were somewhat complicated assays to perform, since *in vitro* preparations of phospholipid spontaneously form micelles which may not accurately mimic the membrane binding properties of intact cells. Nevertheless, similar observations were repeatedly made in a number of model systems and the interpretation still stands.

This situation remained until the beginning of the 1990s when a new form of PLA_2 was discovered [19]. This enzyme was originally purified from cell cytosols and found to be very selective for releasing arachidonic acid from the sn-2 position of phospholipids and is now referred to as cytosolic PLA_2 (hereafter termed $cPLA_2$). This form of PLA_2 was of a higher molecular weight (85–110 kDa) and required only μM concentrations of calcium for activity (i.e., the intracellular concentration). Secondly, the enzyme contained a recognised calcium-dependent membrane binding domain (CalB) such as is found in PKC for example. More significantly perhaps, the activity of $cPLA_2$ was found to be regulated by MAPK-dependent phosphorylation following cell activation. Later work using anti-sense oligonucleotides directed to either $sPLA_2$ or $cPLA_2$ revealed that, in the macrophage, agonist activation of arachidonic acid release was predominantly through the cytosolic form of the enzyme. Indeed, it is now thought that it is $cPLA_2$ which is largely responsible for cellular mediated eicosanoid release and that the phosphorylation mechanism and CalB domain of the protein enable a more responsive control over this process. When enzyme kinetic assays using $cPLA_2$ instead of $sPLA_2$ were used it was found that annexin I was indeed a direct inhibitor of the cytosolic form of the protein at μM concentrations of calcium [20]. It would therefore appear that the natural cellular target for annexin I is $cPLA_2$.

Annexin I is a mediator for the inhibitory action of glucocorticoids on cPLA$_2$ activity

cPLA$_2$ may be activated by increasing intracellular concentrations of calcium resulting in a translocation of the enzyme to plasma membranes. Alternatively, phosphorylation on specific serine residues by MAPK-dependent signal transduction pathways also enhances enzymatic activity. In practice, it is likely that these two processes occur concurrently and have a synergistic effect on arachidonic acid release. However, it is clear from studies using A549 cells that glucocorticoids inhibit only the MAPK-dependent pathway whilst having no effect on calcium mediated effects [10]. A549 cells are a useful model in that they only express the cytosolic form of PLA$_2$ and therefore contributory effects from sPLA$_2$ may be discounted. The activation of cPLA$_2$ by its phosphorylation is revealed electrophoretically by a gel shift assay. In A549 cells this occurs following treatment with EGF or IL-1β, for example. This activation of cPLA$_2$ is inhibited by pre-treatment with glucocorticoids. More importantly, the PLA$_2$ inhibitory effect of glucocorticoids is reversed by neutralising antibodies to annexin I, and, purified recombinant annexin I or short peptide fragments derived from the N-terminus, mimic the action of glucocorticoids [11, 17]. Furthermore, the inhibition of cPLA$_2$ activation by annexin I occurs against a background of no apparent change in COX activity or expression. Taken together, these observations not only re-affirm the original premise that the inhibitory effects of glucocorticoids are mediated *via* the induction of the PLA$_2$ inhibitory protein annexin I, but also indicate a potential mechanism of action. Namely, that an epitope within the N-terminal domain of annexin I interferes somehow with the phosphorylation of cPLA$_2$ and thereby blocks its activation. Clearly, the regulation of either the activity of annexin I, or, its rapid cellular re-distribution following glucocorticoid treatment is central to its inhibitory actions.

The N-terminus of annexin I – a site of regulatory function

Annexin I is a 37 kDa protein, the bulk of which consists of a four-unit repeat structure which has the property of binding phospholipid membranes in a calcium-dependent manner. Each member of the annexin family is distinguished by a unique N-terminal portion of varying lengths. The N-terminal domain of annexin I contains within its sequence several phosphorylation motifs which appear to regulate protein function. Furthermore, the N-terminus also contains sites of interaction with other key proteins. Specifically, the N-terminus of annexin I acts as a substrate for EGF receptor tyrosine kinase and also for for that of the insulin receptor tyrosine kinase (but only after pre-treatment with glucocorticoids) [21, 22]. Phosphorylation of tyrosine 21 lowers the calcium requirement for phospholipid binding and converts tightly associated membrane-bound annexin I to a form whose association with membranes is regulated by calcium as well as promoting its proteolytic degradation [23]. The N-terminus of annexin I is also a substrate for PKC, and phosphorylation of threonine 24, serine 27 and serine 28 inhibits the ability of the protein to aggregate vesicles by raising the calcium requirement for this to occur [24]. Clearly, these mechanisms of phosphorylation (or indeed de-phosphorylation) permit very rapid control over the activity and/or binding properties of annexin I and thereby its cellular disposition.

Residues 1–26 of the N-terminus of annexin I are also involved in vesicle aggregation and this may be mediated by binding to other proteins. In particular residues 1–12 are known to interact with members of the S100 family of proteins [25]. The S100 family comprises a large number of calcium-dependent phospholipid- and cytoskeletal-binding proteins that are ubiquitously expressed but as yet a definitive function for them is unknown. Similarly, residues 13–25 are known to bind strongly cytokeratin 8 and 18 [26] and it may be no coincidence that this same domain also binds to early endosomes (which may contain internalised receptors prior to recycling) [27]. The domain 13–25 also inhibits EGF receptor signaling pathways that lead to activation of cPLA$_2$ [11, 17].

Taken together, these facts may enable us to put together a hypothetical picture of the mobilization of annexin I in cells. This process is depicted in Figure 1. Annexin I in the cytoplasm may reversibly associate with the cell membrane following phosphorylation/de-phosphorylation of the N-terminus by PKC. Once in the membrane compartment, annexin I becomes available for phosphorylation by membrane tyrosine kinases whereupon it remains attached

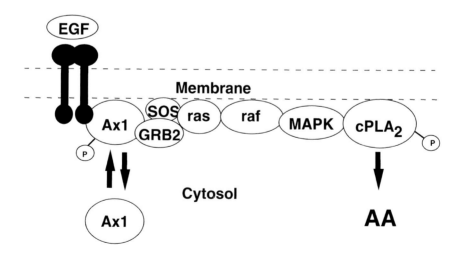

Figure 1. A rapid phosphorylation of cytosolic Ax1 results in translocation to the membrane compartment where recruitment of key signalling intermediates to receptor complexes may be blocked. The activation of downstream kinases is thereby inhibited leading to an inhibition of cvytosolic PLA$_2$ activity.

(and thereby inhibits tyrosine kinase signaling) until proteolysis occurs and the truncated protein is released at the cell surface, and this represents the EDTA-recoverable pool. Clearly, these rapid actions are also influenced by glucocorticoids in a manner that may not require a genomic mechanism operating. Indeed, the activation of phosphatases and/or PKC, focal adhesion kinase and JNK have all been demonstrated to occur rapidly (within minutes) following occupation of the glucocorticoid receptor by its ligand. It remains to be seen whether any of these kinases is responsible for the rapid regulation annexin I activity by glucocorticoids and whether such a process precedes the longer-term genomic-mediated synthesis of annexin I repeatedly observed. However, if proven, such a mechanism would provide an explanation for many facets of annexin I induction. Namely, the complicating effects of serum derived factors and cellular differentiation status, the importance of different cellular pools, and provide a molecular explanation for the rapid glucocorticoid-induced release of annexin I as a distinct event that precedes genomic-mediated induction of protein synthesis.

Conclusions

Since their discovery, the glucocorticoids have traditionally been regarded for their "damping-down" i.e., gene repression activity in controlling inflammation. Whilst this remains a fundamental component of their action, it is now clear that glucocorticoids are also very potent activators of anti-inflammatory mediators of which annexin I is a very important example. In particular, the annexin I-mediated inhibition of PLA_2 activity by glucocorticoids remains a fundamental premise of their action. Despite criticisms from some quarters, there has been no other mechanism elaborated to explain this in the last 20 years of discovery.

References

1 Hamberg M, Svensson J, Samuelsson B (1974) Prostaglandin endoperoxides. A new concept concerning the mode of action and release of prostaglandins. *Proc Natl Acad Sci USA* 71: 3824–3828

2 Vane JR (1971) Inhibition of prostaglandin synthesis as a mechanism of action of aspirin-like drugs. *Nature (New Biol)* 231: 232–235

3 Hong SC, Levine L (1976) Inhibition of arachidonic acid release from cells as the biochemical action of anti-inflammatory steroids. *Proc Natl Acad Sci USA* 73: 1730–1734

4 Flower RJ, Blackwell GJ (1979) Anti-inflammatory steroids induce biosynthesis of a phospholipase A_2 inhibitor which prevents prostaglandin generation. *Nature* 278: 456–459

5 Blackwell GJ, Carnuccio R, Di Rosa M, Flower RJ, Parente L, Persico P (1980) Macrocortin: a polypeptide causing the anti-phospholipase effect of glucocorticoids. *Nature* 287: 147–149

6 Hirata F, Schiffmann E, Venkatasubramanian K, Saloman D, Axelrod J (1980) A phospholipase A_2 inhibitory protein in rabbit neutrophils induced by glucocorticoids. *Proc Natl Acad Sci USA* 77: 2533–2536

7 Russo-Marie F, Duval D (1982) Dexamethasone-induced inhibition of prostaglandin production does not result from a direct action on phospholipase activities but is mediated through a steroid-

inducible factor. *Biochim Biophys Acta* 712: 177–185

8 Solito E, Raugei G, Melli M, Parente L (1991) Dexamethasone induces the expression of the mRNA of annexin I and 2 and the release of annexin I and 5 in differentiated, but not undifferentiated U937 cells. *FEBS Lett* 291: 238–244

9 Croxtall JD, Flower RJ (1992) Lipocortin-1 mediated dexamethasone-induced growth arrest of the A549 lung adenocarcinoma cell line. *Proc Natl Acad Sci USA* 89: 3571–3575

10 Croxtall JD, Choudhury Q, Tokumoto H, Flower RJ (1995) Lipocortin 1 and the control of arachidonic acid release in cell signalling. *Biochem Pharmacol* 50: 465–474

11 Croxtall JD, Choudhury Q, Newman S, Flower RJ (1996) Lipocortin 1 and the control of cPLA$_2$ activity in A549 cells. Glucocorticoids block EGF stimulation of cPLA$_2$ phosphorylation. *Biochem Pharmacol* 52: 351–356

12 Buckingham JC (1996) Stress and the neuroendocrine-immune axis: the pivotal role of glucocorticoids and lipocortin 1. *Brit. J. Pharmacol* 118: 1–1

13 Cirino G, Peers SH, Flower RJ, Browning J, Pepinsky RB (1989) Human recombinant lipocortin 1 has acute local anti-inflammatory properties in the rat paw edema test. *Proc Natl Acad Sci USA* 86: 3428–3432

14 Perretti MP, Flower RJ (1993) Modulation of IL-1 induced neutrophil migration by dexamethasone and lipocortin 1. *J Immunol* 150: 992–999

15 Taylor AD, Cowell AM, Flower RJ, Buckingham JC (1993) Lipocortin 1 mediates an early inhibitory action of glucocorticoids on the secretion of ACTH by the rat anterior pituitary gland *in vitro*. *Neuroendocrinology* 58: 430–439

16 Carey F, Forder R, Edge MD, Greene AR, Horan MA, Strijbos PJLM, Rothwell NJ (1990) Lipocortin-1 modifies pyrogenic actions of cytokines in the rat. *Amer J Physiol* 259: 266–269

17 Croxtall JD, Choudhury Q, Flower RJ (1998) Inhibitory effect of peptides derived from the N-terminus of lipocortin 1 on arachidonic acid release and proliferation in the A549 cell line: identification of E-Q-E-Y-V as a crucial component. *Brit. J. Pharmacol* 123: 975–983

18 Davidson FF, Dennis EA, Powell M, Glenney J (1987) Inhibition of phospholipase A$_2$ by "lipocortins" and calpactins. *J Biol Chem* 262: 1698–1705

19 Diez E, Mong S (1990) Purification of phospholipase A$_2$ from human monocytic leukemic U937 cells. *J Biol Chem* 265: 14654–14661

20 Kim KM, Kim DK, Park YM, Kim C-K, Na DS (1994) Annexin-I inhibits phospholipase A$_2$ by specific interaction, not by substrate depletion. *FEBS Lett* 343: 251–255

21 Pepinsky RB, Sinclair LK (1986) Epidermal growth factor-dependent phosphorylation of lipocortin. *Nature* 321: 81–85

22 Karasik A, Pepinsky RB, Shoelson SE, Kahn CR (1988) Lipocor. *Trends Neurosci* 1 and 2 as substrates for the insulin receptor kinase in rat liver. *J Biol Chem* 263: 11862–11867

23 Schlaepfer DD, Haigler HT (1987) Characterization of Ca^{2+}-dependent phospholipid binding and phosphorylation of lipocortin 1. *J Biol Chem* 262: 6931–6937

24 Schlaepfer DD, Haigler HT (1988) *In vitro* protein kinase C phosphorylation sites of placental lipocortin. *Biochemistry* 27: 4253–4258

25 Seemann J, Weber K, Gerke V (1996) Structural requirements for annexin I-S100C complex-formation. *Biochem J* 319: 123–129

26 Croxtall JD, Wu H-L, Yang H-Y, Smith B, Sutton C, Chang B-I, Shi G-Y, Flower RJ (1998) Lipocortin 1 co-associates with cytokera. *Trends Neurosci* 8 and 18 in A549 cells *via* the N-terminal domain. *Biochim Biophys Acta* 1401: 39–51

27 Seemann J, Weber K, Osborn M, Parton RG, Gerke V (1996) The association of annexin I with early endosomes is regulated by Ca^{2+} and requires an intact N-terminal domain. Mol Biol of the. *Cell* 7: 1359–1374

Glucocorticoids
ed. by N.J. Goulding and R.J. Flower
© 2001 Birkhäuser Verlag/Switzerland

Glucocorticoids and the HPA axis

Anne-Marie Cowell and Julia C. Buckingham

Department of Neuroendocrinology, Division of Neuroscience & Psychological Medicine, Imperial College School of Medicine, Charing Cross Hospital, Fulham Palace Road, London, W6 8RF, UK

Secretion of the glucocorticoids

The glucocorticoids, cortisol and/or corticosterone depending on the species, are steroid hormones produced by cells in the zona fasciculata of the adrenal cortex under the influence of the hypothalamo-pituitary complex (Fig. 1). In normal circumstances their serum concentrations are maintained within narrow limits with pronounced excursions occurring only in accord to a circadian rhythm, which is coupled to the sleep-wake cycle, or in response to physical or emotional stress. The stress-induced changes in circulating glucocorticoids are superimposed upon the existing circadian tone and vary in their rate of onset, magnitude and duration according to the nature, duration and intensity of the insult. For example, insulin-induced hypoglycaemia produces a maximal increase in serum glucocorticoid concentration within 20–30 min and this is followed by a rapid decline in glucocorticoid levels. In contrast, the adrenocortical response to lipopolysaccharide (LPS) emerges only after 1–2 h but usually persists for 24 h or longer. Significant interspecies variations also occur; for example, rats respond very readily to physical stimuli such as cold while humans are particularly sensitive to emotional trauma and pigs show a marked increase in serum cortisol when deprived of food but are relatively unresponsive to many other stimuli (e.g., histamine, cold). Failure to mount an appropriate adrenocortical response to stress is potentially hazardous and indeed disturbances in hypothalamo-pituitary-adrenocortical (HPA) activity are now considered to be a significant contributory factor in the aetiology of various disease processes (see later).

The protective actions of the glucocorticoids

The glucocorticoids exert diverse actions in the body and thereby play a key role in the regulation of crucial homeostatic mechanisms, such as those concerned with metabolic control and immune/inflammatory responses [1, 2]. It is now evident that cortisol/corticosterone display two modes of activity. The

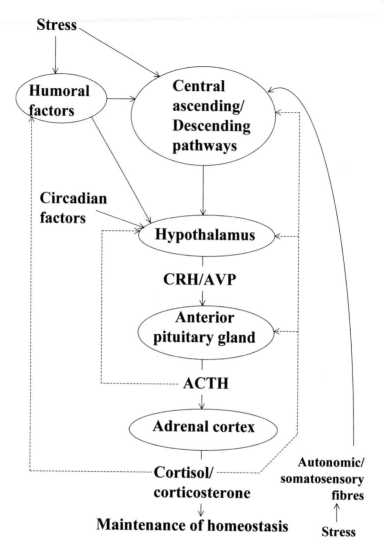

Figure 1. The hypothalamo-pituitary-adrenocortical axis. CRH = corticotrophin releasing hormone; AVP = arginine vasopressin; ACTH = corticotrophin; intact lines = stimulatory influences; dotted lines = inhibitory influences.

first is a "permissive" or "pro-active" role in which the steroids (a) maintain the basal activity of the HPA axis and set its threshold for responding to stress and (b) normalise the body's response to stress by priming the body's defence mechanisms by, for example facilitating the effects of catecholamines on lipid and carbohydrate metabolism (and thereby mobilising energy stores) as well as opposing the actions of insulin (and hence decreasing glucose uptake and utilisation); in addition, the glucocorticoids up-regulate the expression of receptors for inflammatory mediators and act centrally to aid the processes underlying selection attention, integration of sensory information and response selection. The second mode of cortisol/corticosterone action is "suppressive" or "protective" and enables the organism to cope with, adapt to and recover from a stressful insult. Key to this mode are the powerful anti-inflammatory and immunosuppressive actions of the steroids which are attributed to their powerful actions on the growth, differentiation, distribution, function and lifespan of monocytes, macrophages, polymorphonuclear cells and lymphocytes; these prevent the host-defence mechanisms which are activated by stress from overshooting and damaging the organism [3]. Other important protective actions include the ability of the steroids to re-direct metabolism to meet energy demands during stress, to exert important effects within the brain which promote memory processes and to impair non-essential functions such as growth and reproductive function.

The actions of the steroids are effected intracellularly, mainly *via* glucocorticoid receptors (GRs) but also *via* mineralocorticoid receptors (MRs). The MR has a high and approximately equal affinity for the mineralocorticoid, aldosterone, and the endogenous glucocorticoids, corticosterone and cortisol (Kd ~ 1–2 nM). In contrast, the GR is of a lower affinity (Kd cortisol/corticosterone 10–20 nM), does not bind aldosterone readily and is therefore glucocorticoid selective; a truncated form of this receptor, termed GR-β, which does not bind ligand but which has the capacity to bind DNA also exists. Glucocorticoids in the systemic circulation are 95% protein bound, mainly to a specific globulin termed corticosteroid binding globulin (CBG, transcortin) but also to albumin. In principle, only the free steroid has ready access to the intracellular corticosteroid receptors in the target cells. However, local mechanisms which "release" the steroid from its carrier protein(s) appear to exist in at least some target tissues; these include (i) interactions of the carrier protein with cell-surface CBG receptors and (ii) enzymatic cleavage of CBG, for example by serine proteases in inflamed tissues, a process which lowers the affinity of the binding protein for the steroids. Access of the steroids to their receptors is further regulated within the target cells by 11β-hydroxysteroid dehydrogenase (11β-HSD) enzymes which control the interconversion of cortisol/corticosterone to their inactive counterparts, cortisone/11-dehydrocorticosterone [4]. In the kidney type 2 11β-HSD (11β-HSD2), which acts primarily as a dehydrogenase and rapidly inactivates the endogenous glucocorticoids, effectively protects the MRs from cortisol/corticosterone and thus permits selective access of aldosterone to the receptors. MRs in the brain however are not always protected from glucocorticoids in this way and in many instances may be almost fully occupied at low physiological concentrations of cortisol/corticosterone. On the other hand, the delivery of glucocorticoids to GRs in organs such as white adipose tissues and the liver may be facilitated by type 1 11β-HSD (11β-HSD1) which acts primarily as a reductase and thereby regenerates the active steroids from their inactive 11-dehydro metabolites (see the chapter by Feinstein and Schleimer). The permissive actions of the steroids are evident at low physiological concentrations and are mediated at least partially, although probably not exclusively, by the high affinity MR. By contrast, the suppressive or protective actions of the steroids emerge only when cortisol/corticosterone levels are elevated (e.g., by stress) and are effected primarily by the lower affinity GR. The concentration of GRs is known to fluctuate during development, the cell cycle and following disturbances in endocrine status and is an important determinant in cell responsiveness, as is the activity of 11β-HSD enzymes.

Control of glucocorticoid secretion

The hypothalamo-pituitary complex

Cortisol/corticosterone are not stored to any great degree in the adrenal cortex but are synthesised on demand and promptly pass by diffusion across the cell membrane into the systemic circulation. The primary trigger to their synthesis is the 39 amino acid polypeptide hormone, adrenocorticotrophin (ACTH), which is produced in the anterior pituitary gland. ACTH is synthesised in a specialised subgroup of cells, named the corticotrophs, by post-translational cleavage of a large precursor molecule, pro-opiomelanocortin (POMC). POMC also gives rise to a number of other peptides which are co-released with ACTH and are termed collectively the ACTH-related or POMC peptides; these include an N-terminal peptide (N-POMC1-76) of unknown function and β-lipotrophin (β-LPH) which, in turn, may be partially degraded to β-endorphin (which is sometimes used as a marker of ACTH secretion) and γ-LPH. Once released, ACTH acts *via* specific, membrane-bound receptors, termed type 2 melanocortin (MC2) receptors, in the zona fasciculata of the adrenal cortex to activate the conversion of cholesterol to pregnenolone which is the rate-limiting step in the steroidogenic pathway. In addition, it acts on the vasculature to increase adrenal blood flow and thereby aid the passage of the newly synthesised steroids out of the cells into the general systemic circulation. In some circumstances (e.g., adrenal insufficiency) more extensive N-terminal POMC processing may also occur, either within the pituitary gland or at the adrenal level, generating peptides such as N-POMC1-46 and γ-melanocyte-stimulating hormone which appear to augment the steroidogenic capacity of the adrenal cortex by enhancing adrenocortical mitogenesis and potentiating the steroidogenic response to ACTH, respectively.

The release of ACTH from the anterior pituitary gland occurs in an episodic manner mainly under the direction of two hypothalamic neurohormones, a 41 amino acid neuropeptide termed corticotrophin releasing hormone (CRH) and arginine vasopressin (AVP); other hypothalamic factors which may be important in this respect are the pituitary adenylyl cyclase activating peptide (PACAP) which exerts a stimulatory influence and atrial natriuretic peptide (ANP) and substance P, both of which exert inhibitory influences. The frequency of pulses is normally fairly constant over a 24 h period and it is changed in amplitude giving rise to the circadian profile of ACTH and, hence, of glucocorticoid secretion. Increases in pulse amplitude are also responsible for the stress-induced excursions in pituitary-adrenocortical activity although in some instances changes in pulse frequency may also occur.

CRH was first identified in ovine hypothalami by Vale and colleagues [5]; the human peptide was identified subsequently and shown to differ from the ovine peptide by seven amino acids but to be identical to the rat peptide. The CRH gene is well characterised in the rat, mouse and man and is expressed at multiple sites within the central nervous system (CNS; e.g., hypothalamus, amygdala, brain stem) and also in the periphery. CRH destined for the anterior pituitary gland is synthesised in the cell bodies of parvocellular neurones which originate in the paraventricular nucleus (PVN) of the hypothalamus and project to the external lamina of the median eminence. These neurones terminate in close apposition with the capillaries of the hypothalamo-portal complex into which they release their secretory products for transportation to the anterior pituitary gland. The concentration of CRH in hypophyseal portal blood is high (*vs.* peripheral blood) and alters in parallel with perturbations of pituitary-adrenal function (e.g., stress) as does the expression of the peptide and its mRNA in the PVN-median eminence tract. The actions of CRH on the corticotrophs are effected by specific type 1 CRH receptors (CRH-R1) which are positively coupled to adenylyl cyclase *via* a Gs protein [6]; thus stimulation of the receptor causes a rise in intracellular cAMP with subsequent activation of protein kinase A which phosphorylates Ca^{2+} channels, thereby permitting Ca^{2+} influx and the release of ACTH by exocytosis. Activation of CRH-R1 in the pituitary gland also augments POMC gene expression and hence ACTH synthesis and, in the longer term, causes proliferation of the corticotrophs.

The other corticotrophin releasing hormone, AVP shows only weak ACTH-releasing activity *per se*, acting *via* the V1b subclass of AVP receptors which use the phosphatidylinosital signal transduction system. However, AVP potentiates very markedly the corticotrophic responses to CRH and, thus, plays an important role in determining the magnitude of the stress response. Surprisingly, the biochemical basis of this important synergistic response is poorly defined although it is apparent that activation of the V1b receptor potentiates the accumulation of 3'5'-cyclic adenosine monophosphate (3'5'-cAMP) induced by CRH, probably by a mechanism involving protein kinase C-dependent protein phosphorylation. AVP destined for the corticotrophs is derived primarily from a population of CRH-containing parvocellular neurones projecting from the PVN to the median eminence; thus, as for CRH, its concentration in hypophyseal portal blood is relatively high and is further increased by stress. Some AVP may also reach the corticotrophs from magnocellular neurones of the neurohypophyseal system (the primary source of AVP in peripheral blood) *via* the interconnecting short portal vessels. CRH and AVP are co-localised in the same secretory granules within the parvocellular system and may therefore be co-secreted. However, histological studies suggest that in normal circumstances AVP is not expressed by all CRH-positive neurones, thus permitting the ratio of AVP:CRH released to vary in a stimulus-specific manner; equally, not all the corticotrophs express receptors for AVP, thereby permitting another level of control. Although AVP is generally considered to be the second CRH, this is not always the case. For example, in the sheep AVP has precedence over CRH; similarly in rodents and possibly in man, AVP appears to be the dominant factor driving ACTH release in conditions of repeated or sustained stress (see later).

Stress induced activation of the hypothalamus

The parvocellular CRH/AVP neurones in the hypothalamus receive inputs from many ascending and descending nervous pathways [2]; in addition they are sensitive to a variety of substances which may be borne by the blood or the cerebrospinal fluid (e.g., glucose, steroids) and to local factors released from glial cells or interneurones (e.g., eicosanoids, cytokines). Major roles have been identified for (a) pathways projecting to the PVN from the prefrontal cortex and the limbic system (hippocampus, amygdala, lateral septum and the bed nucleus of the stria terminalis, BNST) and (b) inputs from the brain stem nuclei, in particular the nucleus tractus solitarius (NTS), which relay sensory information directly to the PVN and other parts of the brain; other pathways, for example those arising from the raphe nuclei, are also likely to contribute. The precise complement of neural pathways, humoral substances and local mediators which orchestrates the release of CRH/AVP in stress almost certainly depends upon the nature of the stimulus and the status of the individual at the time of the stress, but some classification according to the type of stress is now possible [7]. For example, visceral "homeostatic" stressors which lack a cognitive component (e.g., acute hypotension) initiate HPA responses by activating afferents fibres which signal *via* the brain stem nuclei and the noradrenergic pathways which project from the brain stem to the PVN; the responses to some homeostatic stressors also involve humoral mechanisms, for example the responses to hypertonicity and hypoglycaemia involve intrahypothalamic osmotic- and glucose-sensitive neurones respectively. Visceral stressors with a significant cognitive component, for example footshock restraint, or cold, utilise somatosensory afferents and central pathways involving both the brain stem nuclei and cortical-limbic system to activate the PVN. The cortical-limbic system also plays a fundamental role in effecting the HPA responses to emotional stressors; the role of the amygdala, a key area in co-ordinating the behavioural, autonomic and neuroendocrine responses to fear or anxiety, is well documented in this regard as too is the importance of the hippocampus which is critical to cognitive function, in particular learning and memory.

Challenges to the host-defence system, such as those provoked by infection, injury or inflammation, pose a major threat to homeostasis and thus constitute a severe stress. Not surprisingly, in experimental animals and in man such insults result in a marked increase in the activity of the HPA axis. There is now unequivocal evidence that this response is mediated primarily by the army of products (e.g., interleukins, eicosanoids, histamine, phospholipase A_2) released from the activated immune/inflammatory cells [2, 7–9]. The mechanisms by which these agents increase glucocorticoid secretion are complex and varied. Some of these substances may influence the HPA axis directly, acting mainly at the hypothalamic level to stimulate CRH/AVP release but also on the anterior pituitary gland and adrenal cortex to augment or sustain the adrenocortical response. Others may act locally at the site of the infection or inflammatory lesion to stimulate sensory fibres and thereby activate the central pathways which precipitate CRH/AVP release. In addition, many of the mediators provoke widespread pathological effects in the body (e.g., hypotension, hypoglycaemia) which themselves will stimulate the axis by the mechanisms outlined above.

The cytokines, interleukin-1β (IL-1β) and IL-6, are particularly important in initiating the HPA response to bacterial and viral infections and much research has focused on the mechanism whereby they activate the HPA axis [2, 7–9]. The main mechanisms which have been proposed to explain their actions are:

a) The cytokines act directly on the PVN to stimulate CRH release *via* a mechanism dependent on prostanoid generation. This has been refuted on the basis that the cytokines, which are large polypeptides (17–26 kDa), are unlikely to penetrate the blood-brain barrier and thereby gain access to their targets. However, the possibility that the cytokines enter the brain *via* (i) fenestrated regions of the barrier (e.g., *organum vasculosum lamina terminalis*, OVLT), (ii) areas in which the permeability is increased (e.g., by local inflammation) or (iii) a specific transporter system cannot be ruled out.

b) The cytokines act on the specialised endothelial cells of the blood brain barrier itself and cause the release of soluble mediators, particularly eicosanoids, which may trigger CRH/AVP release by a variety of these mechanisms; these include activation of neural pathways and/or induction of *de novo* synthesis of cytokines in the hypothalamus and elsewhere in the brain, which are required to drive the HPA response. The presence of IL-1 receptors on endothelial cells and the increase in IL-1 mRNA expression observed in the hypothalamus and other brain areas of rodents challenged with endotoxin support this concept.

c) The hypothalamic responses to peripheral cytokines involve the sequential activation of sensory fibres, brain stem nuclei (notably the NTS) and the ventral noradrenergic pathways (and possibly others) to the PVN. This view concurs with the findings that the expression of IL-1β mRNA in the hypothalamus and the hypersecretion of ACTH release induced by intraperitoneal injection of endotoxin or IL-1β are ablated by sub-diaphragmatic vagotomy and that C-fibres are required to initiate the HPA responses to local inflammatory lesions induced by turpentine [9]. However, it is at odds with reports that cytokines activate the NTS, and hence the connections between the NTS and the PVN, by mechanisms that are independent of the vagus but which may involve local prostanoid-dependent interactions with the blood brain barrier.

Negative feedback control of the HPA axis

The adrenocortical responses to incoming stimuli are tightly controlled by the glucocorticoids and the other hormones of the HPA axis. Thus the POMC derived peptides, ACTH and β-endorphin, both inhibit the secretion of CRH/AVP by the hypothalamus, probably *via* actions at the level of the median eminence since neither peptide readily penetrates the blood brain barrier. In addition, ultra-short loop feedback actions have been attributed to both CRH and AVP; the physiological significance of these actions is unclear and more recent data suggest that CRH may exert a positive effect on its own secretion. Most important however are the powerful inhibitory influences exerted by the glucocorticoids on the secretion of CRH/AVP and ACTH by the hypothalamus and anterior pituitary gland respectively [10–12]. Thus, elevations in circulating glucocorticoid levels brought about for example by adrenal tumours or administration of exogenous steroids effectively suppress the circadian rise in pituitary-adrenocortical activity and the HPA responses to stress. Conversely, there is a sustained hypersecretion of ACTH and an exaggerated ACTH response to stress in subjects with adrenocortical insufficiency (e.g., Addison's disease) which is corrected by glucocorticoid replacement therapy. The feedback actions of the steroids are extremely complex as they are exerted at multiple sites within the axis and involve multiple molecular mechanisms which operate over three time domains; these are termed the rapid (or fast), early delayed and late delayed phases of feedback inhibition.

Phases of glucocorticoid feedback

Rapid feedback occurs within 2–3 min of an increase in glucocorticoid levels. It is of short duration (<10 min) and is followed by a "silent" period during which the ACTH response to stress is unimpaired even though the circulating steroid levels may still be elevated. Rapid feedback is sensitive to the rate of change rather than the absolute concentration of steroid in the blood and may therefore provide an important means whereby the HPA response to stress is terminated; alternatively, it may serve to blunt the responses to a second stress incurred at a time when the steroid levels are still rising in response to the first stress. The early delayed phase of feedback develops approximately 0.5–2 h after an acute elevation in plasma steroid levels. Its is normally maximal within 2–4 h and, depending on the intensity of the stimulus, may persist for up to 24 h. Both the circadian and stress-induced excursions in ACTH secretion are suppressed with an intensity that is directly proportional to the concentration of steroid previously reached in the blood. Late delayed feedback, which has a latency of about 24 h, develops only after a very substantial rise in steroid levels and is frequently the consequence of repeated or continuous administration of high doses of corticosteroids. It may persist for days or weeks after the steroid treatment is withdrawn and is thus largely responsible for the potentially life-threatening suppression of the HPA axis associated with abrupt cessation of long-term treatment with high doses of steroids in, for example, rheumatoid arthritis.

Mechanisms of glucocorticoid feedback

The rapid feedback actions of the glucocorticoids are exerted primarily at the hypothalamic level; weaker actions also occur at the pituitary level but the contribution, if any, of extrahypothalamic sites in the CNS is ill-defined. The underlying molecular mechanisms are poorly understood but the effects are too rapid to be dependent on the genomic actions of the glucocorticoids mediated *via* intracellular MRs or GRs. Although there are some reports to the contrary, the majority of data suggest that the rapid actions of the steroids may be mediated by novel non-classical steroid receptors located close to or within cell membranes which, when activated, cause membrane stabilization and inhibit exocytosis, possibly by blocking Ca^{2+} influx. The early and late delayed phases of glucocorticoid feedback inhibition by contrast are mediated by classical intracellular corticosteroid receptors located primarily in the anterior pituitary gland, the hypothalamus and the hippocampus, but also elsewhere in the brain. Both the high affinity MRs and the lower affinity GRs are involved. Current evidence suggests that MR (located predominantly in the hippocampus) may maintain the tonic inhibitory influence of steroids on HPA function in non-stress conditions as these receptors, which are not "protected" by 11 β-HSD, are normally almost fully occupied by glucocorticoids even at the nadir of the circadian rhythm [13]. GRs on the other hand are extensively occupied only when the glucocorticoid level is raised for example by stress, disease or administration of exogenous steroids and thus serve to restore glucocorticoid release to basal level. Cortisol/corticosterone preferentially target the brain and terminate the HPA response to stress primarily through GRs in the parvocellular PVN and possibly in other brain areas whilst exogenous synthetic glucocorticoids such as dexamethasone which have limited access to the brain act predominantly at the pituitary level to block stress-induced HPA activity [13].

Early delayed feedback requires *de novo* generation of protein second messengers which serve to inhibit the release of ACTH and its hypothalamic releasing factors; several proteins are likely to be involved including annexin 1 (ANX-1, lipocortin 1), a 37 kDa member of the annexin family of Ca^{2+} and phospholipid binding proteins (see below). The genes encoding POMC in the pituitary gland and CRH/AVP in the parvocellular PVN neurones may also be repressed during the early delayed phase of feedback; however, the consequent down-regulation of ACTH, CRH and AVP synthesis emerges relatively slowly and, with existing techniques, is not normally discernible until some hours after the onset of inhibition of peptide release. Late delayed feedback is characterised by inhibition of the synthesis and the release of CRH/AVP and ACTH in the hypothalamus and anterior pituitary gland respectively. The inhibition of synthesis again reflects the inhibitory influence of the steroids on the genes encoding each of the three peptides but the concomitant inhibition of peptide release cannot be explained fully in this way as peptide stores are rarely fully depleted. Reductions in the pools available for release is a possible explanation but the underlying molecular mechanisms await elucidation.

Role of annexin 1 in early delayed glucocorticoid feedback

Annexin 1 was first identified in rat peritoneal macrophages where it was shown to be glucocorticoid-inducible and to contribute to the powerful anti-inflammatory and immunosuppressive actions of the steroids [14]. More recently substantial amounts of ANX-1 mRNA and protein have also been detected in the cells of the neuroendocrine system. The protein is particularly abundant in the anterior pituitary gland and in areas of the hypothalamus associated with the regulation of anterior pituitary function (i.e., the median eminence and PVN) but is also expressed in lesser amounts elsewhere in the brain (e.g., cortex, hippocampus). In these tissues, as in several peripheral cell/tissues, glucocorticoids regulate both the expression and the subcellular distribution of ANX-1. Thus, both *in vitro* and *in vivo* glucocorticoids induce *de novo* synthesis of ANX-1 and promote the exportation of the intracellular protein to the outer cell surface (pericellular pool) where it is retained by a Ca^{2+}-dependent mechanism [11, 14–17].

It is now known that ANX-1 fulfils a significant role as a mediator of glucocorticoid action in the HPA axis, acting mainly at the levels of the hypothalamus and anterior pituitary gland but also possibly at other sites in the brain (e.g., hippocampus) to effect the negative feedback actions of the steroids on the axis. In the rat *in vivo* central (i.c.v.) or peripheral (s.c.) administration of anti-ANX-1 anti-sera effectively reverses the ability of glucocorticoids (corticosterone or dexamethasone) to block the increases in ACTH and corticosterone secretion induced by central (i.c.v.) or peripheral (i.p.) injection of IL-1β [11, 16]. Conversely, central injections of the full length human recombinant ANX-1 (hu-r-ANX-1) or the N-terminal peptides, ANX-1$_{1-188}$ and ANX-1$_{Ac2-26}$, abolish the rises in glucocorticoid secretion induced by central injections of either IL-1β or IL-6 [15]. Data from *in vitro* studies indicate that ANX-1 contributes to the actions of the steroids within both the hypothalamus and the anterior pituitary gland. Thus, at the hypothalamic level the inhibitory actions of glucocorticoids on the release of CRH/AVP provoked by IL-1α and β, IL-6 or IL-8 are mimicked by hrANX-1$_{1-346}$ and ANX-1$_{1-188}$ and reversed by a neutralising anti-ANX-1 antibody [16]. Similarly, like the glucocorticoids, hrANX-1$_{1-346}$ and ANX-1$_{1-188}$ suppress the secretagogue-driven release of ACTH from pituitary tissue *in vitro* [11, 18]. Moreover, the responses to dexamethasone are reversed specifically by anti-ANX-1 antisera and ANX-1 antisense oligodeoxynucleotides (ODNs) directed against sequences specific to the ANX-1 mRNA [18, 19].

It is not yet known how ANX-1 exerts its inhibitory actions on peptide release. However, three lines of evidence support the proposal that the prompt exportation of ANX-1 from cells induced by the steroid is critical in this regard, possibly because it enables the protein to gain access to cell surface binding sites (putative receptors). Firstly, on a temporal basis, the manifestation of steroid-induced inhibition of peptide release parallels the exportation of ANX-1, both being evident with 15 min and maximal by 90 min of a steroid challenge [11, 17, 18]. Secondly, the inhibitory actions of the steroids on peptide release are abolished by processes which inhibit the cellular exportation of ANX-1 (protein synthesis inhibitors, ANX-1 antisense oligonucleotides) [18, 19] Thirdly, the antisera which so effectively abrogate the inhibitory actions of glucocorticoids on peptide release *in vivo* and *in vitro* would be unlikely to penetrate cells rapidly but could readily sequester ANX-1 at a pericellular site; similarly, exogenous hrANX-1$_{1-346}$ and ANX-1$_{1-188}$ would reach cell surface "receptors" more readily than intracellular targets. Using a combination of fluorescence activated cell (FAC) analysis/sorting and electron microscopy, we have identified saturable, high affinity ANX-1 binding sites on the surface of several anterior pituitary cell types, including corticotrophs; the binding is Ca^{2+}- and temperature sensitive [20]. Evidence that the binding sites serve as receptors derives from the Kd (~10 nM) which is indicative of a putative receptor and from the fact that ablation of the binding sites (with trypsin) destroys the ability of anti-ANX-1 antisera to abrogate the inhibitory actions of dexamethasone on ACTH release [20]. Moreover, when viewed by fluorescence or confocal microscopy, the distribution of the binding sites on the cell surface appears punctate; this pattern is consistent with the widespread phenomenon of ligand-induced receptor clustering, a process which may be essential for internalisation [20].

In principal, ANX-1 could act as an autocrine agent, binding to and acting on the cells from which it is released; alternatively, it could act as a paracrine agent, modulating the activity of adjacent cells. Studies based on immunohistochemistry [21] and FAC analysis/sorting in permeabilised pituitary cells [22] have shown that in the adenohypophysis ANX-1 is expressed by both endocrine (e.g., corticotrophs) and non-secretory (e.g., folliculostellate) cells but that it is particularly abundant in the latter. Similarly, the majority of data indicate that in the brain ANX-1 is normally more abundant in glial cells (in particular microglia) than neurones but that following brain injury it is also expressed in substantial amounts by astrocytes and by invading leukocytes

[14]. Taken together, these findings suggest that ANX-1 originates primarily from cells of glial or immunological lineage in the brain/neuroendocrine system; they thus raise the possibility that, by serving as a paracrine agent, ANX-1 acts as an important mediator of neuroendocrine-immune communication providing a means whereby not only resident glia and glia-like cells but also migrating/infiltrating steroid sensitive immune/inflammatory cells (e.g., macrophages) may modulate peptide release and thus help to contain the neuroendocrine responses to immune insults [11, 14, 21].

Glucocorticoid secretion in repeated or sustained stress

The majority of studies on stress and HPA function have focused on acute stresses and relatively little is known of either the characteristics or the mechanisms controlling the HPA responses to repeated or sustained stress (for detailed review see [23]). Such conditions are of course inherent to our lifestyle and environment and a deeper understanding of their influence on neuroendocrine function is thus highly desirable, particularly as prolonged elevations in circulating corticosteroids are potentially harmful and may contribute to the pathogenesis of a wide range of disorders (see later). However, for both ethical and practical reasons it is difficult to develop appropriate animal models and the data available suggest that the HPA responses observed depend upon both the nature of the stress and the species.

In some cases, the HPA responses to repeated (successive or intermittent) or sustained (chronic) stressful stimuli are attenuated. For example, "tolerance" develops to stresses such as cold, handling, saline injection or water deprivation (induced by replacement of drinking water with physiological saline). Some degree of "cross tolerance" may occur between stresses which invoke similar pathways/mechanisms to increase CRH/AVP release. Thus, for example, repeated handling reduces the subsequent adrenocortical response to a saline injection; however, rats tolerant to the C-fibre dependent stress of exposure to a cold environment, respond to the novel stress of immobilisation with a normal or even enhanced rise in serum corticosterone. In other situations however tolerance does not develop; thus, the HPA responses to the intermittent stresses of electric foot shock, insulin hypoglycaemia or IL-1β and those to the chronic stress of septicaemia are maintained or even enhanced.

The sustained release of ACTH in repeated/chronic stress appears to be driven mainly by AVP. Thus, in rats subjected to repetitive foot shock, brain surgery or injection of IL-1β/LPS, AVP is synthesised in and released from the parvocellular neurones in the PVN in preference to CRH [23]; in addition, the sensitivity of the pituitary gland to AVP is well maintained while that to CRH is reduced. Similarly, the expression of AVP but not CRH in the parvocellular PVN is increased in rats with experimentally induced arthritis; moreover, while the arthritic rats respond to LPS with a rise ACTH secretion, they are relatively unresponsive to a novel neurogenic stress normally driven mainly by

CRH. The "switch" to AVP as the principal driving force to the corticotrophs in repetitive/chronic stress may reflect disruption of the negative feedback action of the glucocorticoids for the expression of MR in the hippocampus and GR in the PVN is reduced in conditions of chronic stress.

The stress response during development

The glucocorticoids fulfil complex organisational effects both pre- and post-natally and, thus, play a key role in "developmental programming". It is not surprising, therefore, that the HPA axis is tightly regulated during perinatal life. In the later stages of gestation the foetus secretes substantial quantities of cortisol/corticosterone and also responds to stress with an increase in HPA activity which is sensitive to the negative feedback actions of the glucocorti-coids. Paradoxically, however, in rodents HPA function regresses postnatally and a period ensues during which the HPA response to stress is attenuated. In the rat, this stress hyporesponsive phase (SHRP) normally persists from post-natal day 5 (P5) to P14, although a mature stress response to some stimuli may not emerge for up to 5–6 weeks. Since the SHRP coincides with an important phase of development, it seems likely that it may serve to protect the organism from the potentially harmful effects of overexposure to glucocorticoids. However, the refractoriness of the HPA axis to stress in the SHRP is not absolute and in certain cases it may be at least partially overridden. For exam-ple, modest rises in serum ACTH and corticosterone are elicited by IL-1β, hypoglycaemia, glutamate and histamine throughout this period. Exceptionally, the hypersecretion of ACTH provoked by LPS in the SHRP matches that observed in the adult although the associated rise in serum corti-costerone does not; moreover, paradoxically, both the ACTH and the corticos-terone responses to kainic acid are more robust at P12 than P18. These and many other data suggest that the processes involved in the maturation of the stress response are complex and stimulus dependent. They are therefore likely to involve a variety of factors which act in concert at different levels of the axis during the developmental period. These include immaturity of the neural and humoral mechanisms effecting the release of CRH/AVP in stress, impairment of the synergy between CRH and AVP and enhanced sensitivity of the axis to the regulatory actions of the glucocorticoids [24].

Despite its tight control, the developing HPA axis shows a high degree of plasticity and a growing body of evidence suggests that disturbances in the glucocorticoid milieu or exposure to factors which influence the expression of the glucocorticoid receptors at critical stages of development may (a) trigger a plethora of pathologies (e.g., growth retardation, impairment of CNS develop-ment) and (b) precipitate abnormalities in glucocorticoid secretion which per-sist into adult life and may increase the susceptibility of the individual to con-ditions as diverse as hypertension, insulin resistance, cognitive and other behavioural disorders and allergic/inflammatory disease. Perinatal manipulations which alter GR (but not MR) expression in the brain are particularly hazardous in this regard as, by disrupting the negative feedback mechanisms, they alter the responsivity of the HPA axis to stress throughout the lifetime of the individual [13]. For example, exposure of neonatal rats to exogenous glucocorticoids or stimuli which raise serum glucocorticoids (e.g., injection of LPS) results in the adult in down regulation of GR in the hippocampus and hypothalamus, reduced sensitivity of the HPA axis to the negative feedback actions of the glucocorticoids and exaggerated HPA responses to stress. Similar long-term changes in GR expression and HPA function occur in rats subjected to prolonged periods of maternal separation and are associated with alterations in T-cell antibody responses and in the incidence of age-related neuropathies. Conversely, neonatal handling, which increases hippocampal GR expression by mechanisms involving serotonin, reduces the magnitude and duration of the stress response in the adult; maternal care may therefore help to programme events which regulate responses to stress in the adult and, thus, reduce vulnerability to disease.

Sexual dimorphism in HPA function

In adults, distinct sexually dimorphic patterns of glucocorticoid secretion emerge. Serum glucocorticoid concentrations are consistently higher in the female than the male with further increases occurring towards the middle of the menstrual/oestrous cycle just prior to ovulation and in the late stages of pregnancy. These changes are due partly to the positive effects of oestrogen on the expression of CBG. In addition, oestrogen exerts significant effects at the hypothalamic level increasing the synthesis and the release of CRH, a phenomenon which may be implicated in the aetiology of the relatively high incidence of emotional disorders (e.g., depression, anxiety) in the female which are characterised by enhanced CRH secretion [25]. Further modulation may be brought about by progesterone which, when present in large amounts (e.g., in the pre-menstrual phase or pregnancy), binds readily to but is only weakly active at mineralocorticoid receptors in the hippocampus [26].

Stress responses in the ageing

In both sexes, the serum glucocorticoid concentrations tend to increase in ageing individuals, particularly in disease states; in addition, although sometimes delayed, the HPA responses to stress are frequently exaggerated and prolonged [13]. This "ageing" process has been attributed in part to down-regulation of the corticosteroid receptors (GR and MR) in the hippocampus and hypothalamus and the consequent emergence of a resistance of the HPA axis to the negative feedback actions of the glucocorticoids. The consequences are potentially important for hyperglucocorticoidaemia is considered to be an important contributory factor to a number of age-related diseases, including neurodegenerative conditions, cognitive dysfunction, osteoporosis, non-insulin dependent diabetes mellitus, hypertension and other cardiovascular disease, and the decline in immunocompetence.

Increasing evidence suggests that sustained elevations in serum glucocorticoids, such as those that occur in chronic stress, may contribute to the processes of neurodegeneration; for example, cortisol levels correlate with mental deterioration and decreased hippocampal volume in individuals suffering from Alzheimer's disease [13]. The toxic actions of the steroids, which have been studied most widely in the hippocampus, are associated with altered glutaminergic transmission, a long-term enhancement of Ca^{2+} influx and depletion of ATP stores with consequent impairment of essential energy-requiring processes such as glucose uptake. The vulnerability of the neurones may be further enhanced by a reduction in neurotrophic capacity for elevations in serum glucocorticoids induced by chronic stress or administration of exogenous steroids inhibit the expression of brain derived neurotrophic factor mRNA and also tyrosine kinase which is required for growth factor action.

Effects of glucocorticoids on cognitive function and mood

Glucocorticoids released in stress may exert significant effects on cognitive function, mood and behaviour and the reception of sensory inputs. Subjects whose serum glucocorticoids are raised due to either Cushing's disease or exogenous steroids also show marked disturbances in sleep with a reduction in time spent in the rapid eye movement (REM) phase.

Studies on laboratory animals have shown that glucocorticoids act in the neocortex and limbic system (hippocampus, septum, amygdala) to modify learning and memory processes in a context-dependent manner. Thus, an acute rise in glucocorticoids may facilitate learning and memory processes but also eliminate learned behaviour that is no longer of relevance. The complex actions of the steroids involve both MR and GR, with MR effecting the appraisal of information and response selection and GR promoting the processes underlying the consolidation of acquired information. The long-term effects of glucocorticoids on learning and memory are less well researched and the data available are conflicting. However, a correlation between impaired cognitive function/reduced volume of hippocampal formation and average plasma cortisol levels in Cushing's patients has been reported. Similarly, elderly individuals who developed hypercortisolism over a period of 4 years showed deficits in long-term memory [13].

Raised glucocorticoid levels have also been implicated in the aetiology of depression (although, paradoxically, patients with adrenal insufficiency also often experience depression). Thus approximately half of patients with iatrogenic or endogenous Cushing's disease show psychological disturbances of which depression is the most common; some subjects show euphoric or manic behaviour and, in some cases, overt psychoses. Alternatively, 50% of patients suffering from depression have a hyperactive HPA system which is associated with adrenal hypertrophy and enhanced CRH/AVP expression in the PVN. These patients also show steroid feedback resistance at the level of the PVN and the anterior pituitary gland; this may be due to an imbalance of MR/GR expression or function since tricyclic anti-depressants increase the expression of corticosteroid receptors, particularly MR, in the brain in parallel with normalisation of HPA tone whilst systemic administration of anti-mineralocorticoids impairs the therapeutic efficacy of anti-depressants [13].

Disorders associated with a reduction in HPA activity

Adrenocortical insufficiency precipitates a vulnerability to stress and increases susceptibility to infection as well as to various autoimmune, inflammatory and allergic disorders. In addition, a reduction in HPA activity appears to be a vulnerability factor for post-traumatic stress syndrome, chronic fatigue syndrome and fibromyalgia. Thus post-traumatic stress syndrome is characterised by enhanced glucocorticoid feedback, perhaps through hippocampal MRs, whilst chronic fatigue syndrome and fibromyalgia seem to be associated with deficient CRH function and reduced adrenocortical sensitivity respectively [13].

References

1　Buckingham JC (2000) Glucocorticoids: role in stress of. *In*: G Fink (ed.): *The encyclopaedia of stress*. Academic Press, New York, 261–279

2　Buckingham JC, Christian HC, Gillies GE, Philip JG, Taylor AD (1996) The hypothalamo-pituitary-adrenocortical immune axis. *In*: JA Marsh, MD Kendall (eds): *The physiology of immunity*. CRC Press, Boca Raton, 331–354

3　Munck A, Guyre PM, Holbrook NJ (1984) Physiological functions of glucocorticoids and their relation to pharmacological actions. *Endocrin Rev* 51: 25–44

4　Seckl JR (1997) 11β-hydroxysteroid dehydrogenase in the brain: a novel regulator of glucocorticoid action? *Frontiers Neuroendocrinol* 18: 49–99

5　Vale W, Spiess J, Rivier L, Rivier J (1981) Characterisation of a 41-residue ovine hypothalamic peptide that stimulates secretion of corticotropin and β-endorphin. *Science* 213: 1394–1397

6　Chalmers DT, Lovenberg TW, Grigoriadis DE, Behan DP, De Sousa EB (1996) Corticotrophin-releasing factor receptors: from biology to drug design. *Trends Pharmacol Sci* 17: 166–172

7　Buckingham JC, Loxley HD, Christian HC, Philip JG (1996) Activation of the HPA axis by immune insults; roles and interactions of cytokines, eicosanoids, and glucocorticoids. *Pharmacol Biochem Behav* 54: 285–298

8　Turnbull A, Rivier C (1999) Regulation of the hypothalamic-pituitary-adrenal axis by cytokines: actions and mechanisms of action. *Physiol Rev* 79: 1–71

9　Mulla A, Buckingham JC (1999) Regulation of the hypothalamo-pituitary-adrenal axis by cytokines. *In*: M Harbuz (ed.): *Stress and immunity: The neuroendocrine link*. Balliere's. *Clin Endocrinol* 13: 503–522

10　Keller-Wood ME, Dallman MF (1984) Corticosteroid inhibition of ACTH secretion. *Endocrin Rev* 5: 1–25

11 Buckingham JC (1996) Stress and the neuroendocrine immune axis: the pivotal role of glucocorticoids and lipocortin 1. *Brit J Pharmacol* 118: 1–19

12 Buckingham JC, Smith T, Loxley HD (1992) The control of ACTH secretion. *In*: VHT James (ed.): *The adrenal cortex*. Raven Press, New York, 131–158

13 de Kloet ER, Vreugdenhil E, Citzl MS, Joels M (1998) Brain corticosteroid receptor balance in health and disease. *Endocrin Rev* 19: 269–301

14 Ahluwalia A, Buckingham JC, Croxtall JD, Flower RJ, Goulding NJ, Perretti M (1996) The Biology of Annexin 1. *In*: BA Seaton (ed.): *The annexins*. R Landes and Co, Austin, 161–199

15 Loxley HD, Cowell AM, Flower RJ, Buckingham JC (1993) Modulation of the hypothalamo-pituitary-adrenocortical responses to cytokines in the rat by lipocortin 1 and glucocorticoids: a role for lipocortin 1 in the feedback inhibition of CRF-41 release? *Neuroendocrinology* 57: 801–813

16 Taylor AD, Loxley HD, Flower RJ, Buckingham JC (1995) Immunoneutralization of lipocortin 1 reverses the inhibitory effects of dexamethasone on cytokine-induced hypothalamo-pituitary-adrenocortical activity *in vitro* and *in vivo*. *Neuroendocrinology* 62: 19–31

17 Philip JG, Flower RJ, Buckingham JC (1998) Blockade of the classical pathway of protein secretion does not affect the cellular exportation of lipocortin 1. *Reg Peptides* 73: 133–139

18 Taylor AD, Cowell AM, Flower RJ, Buckingham JC (1993) Lipocortin 1 mediates an early inhibitory action of glucocorticoids on the secretion of ACTH by the rat anterior pituitary gland *in vitro*. *Neuroendocrinology* 58: 430–439

19 Taylor AD, Christian HC, Morris JF, Flower RJ, Buckingham JC (1997) An antisense oligodeoxynucleotide to lipocortin 1 reverses the inhibitory actions of dexamethasone on the release of adrenocorticotropin from rat pituitary tissue *in vitro*. *Endocrinology* 138: 2909–2918

20 Christian HC, Taylor AD, Flower RJ, Morris JF, Buckingham JC (1997) Characterization and localization of lipocortin 1-binding sites on rat anterior pituitary cells by fluorescence-activated cell analysis/sorting and electron microscopy. *Endocrinology* 138: 5341–5351

21 Traverso VT, Christian HC, Morris JF, Buckingham JC (1999) Lipocortin 1 (annexin 1) is localised in pituitary folliculostellate cells. *Endocrinology* 140: 4311–4319

22 Christian HC, Flower RJ, Morris JF, Buckingham JC (1999) Localisation and semi-quantitative measurement of lipocortin 1 in rat anterior pituitary cells by fluorescence activated cell analysis/sorting and electron microscopy. *J Neuroendocrinol* 11: 707–714

23 Aguilera G (1994) Regulation of pituitary ACTH release during chronic stress. *Frontiers Neuroendocrinol* 15: 321–350

24 Rosenfeld P, Suchecki AJ, Levine S (1992) Multifactorial regulation of the hypothalamic-pituitary-adrenal axis during development. *Neurosci Behav Rev* 129: 384–388

25 Vamvakopoulos NC, Chrousos GP (1994) Hormonal regulation of human corticotropin releasing hormone gene expression: implications for the sexual dimorphism of the stress response and immune inflmmatory reaction. *Endocrin Rev* 15: 409–420

26 de Kloet ER, Rotd NY, van den Berg DTW, Oitzl MS (1994) Brain mineralocorticoid receptor function. *Ann N Y Acad Sci* 746: 8–21

The role of 11β-hydroxysteroid dehydrogenase in regulating glucocorticoid action

Marc B. Feinstein and Robert P. Schleimer

Johns Hopkins Asthma and Allergy Center, 5501 Hopkins Bayview Circle, Baltimore, MD 21224-6801, USA

Introduction

The activity of hydrocortisone, the major endogenous glucocorticoid in humans, is determined at multiple levels along a complex metabolic pathway that begins with the release of corticotropin releasing hormone (CRH) at the hypothalamus and ends in the nucleus of target cells where the activated glucocorticoid receptor regulates cellular functions. Modulation of glucocorticoid synthesis by the hypothalamic-pituitary-adrenal axis is described in detail in the chapter by Cowell and Buckingham. This chapter will examine how the activity of hydrocortisone may be controlled locally in various target tissues by the enzyme 11β-hydroxysteroid dehydrogenase (11β-HSD).

11β-HSD is a principal pathway for the metabolism of hydrocortisone, reversibly converting it to the inactive glucocorticoid cortisone through oxidation of the C-11 hydroxyl group to its ketone counterpart (Fig. 1). This enzyme can play an important role in modulating endogenous glucocorticoid activity by regulating the amount of hydrocortisone available to bind the glucocorticoid receptor. Inhibitors of this enzyme have long been known to possess anti-inflammatory properties. Extracts of licorice, for example, which contain the

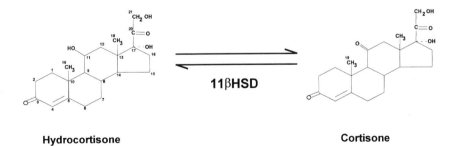

Hydrocortisone   **11βHSD**   **Cortisone**

Figure 1. Interconversion of hydrocortisone and cortisone by 11β-HSD.

potent 11β-HSD inhibitor glycyrrhetinic acid, were first advocated as an asthma treatment by the Greek botanist Theophrastus (370–288 B.C.) [1]. These remain a popular asthma treatment today in China and its Far Eastern neighbors. More recently, glycyrrhetinic acid has been used to treat a number of other ailments, including Addison's Disease and rheumatoid arthritis. Although structurally similar to glucocorticoids, glycyrrhetinic acid binds to the glucocorticoid receptor weakly; its affinity is several orders of magnitude less than that of hydrocortisone. Moreover, the efficacy of glycyrrhetinic acid in Addison's disease requires the presence of either a functioning adrenal gland or the administration of exogenous glucocorticoids. These were some of the early observations which suggested that glycyrrhetinic acid does not act through the glucocorticoid receptor but rather by potentiating the activity of glucocorticoids already present through 11β-HSD inactivation.

Biochemical properties of 11β-HSD

The involvement of 11β-HSD in such a wide diversity of physiologic processes is made possible by the presence of multiple proteins with 11β-HSD activity. Two forms of the 11β-HSD enzyme have been cloned and sequenced thus far and others are suspected. 11β-HSD Type 1 (11β-HSD$_1$), also called the liver isoform, has a K_m for hydrocortisone in the range of normal circulating glucocorticoid levels, about 1 μm. It requires NADP as a cofactor and is a bidirectional enzyme. Northern blot studies in rat tissues have found that 11β-HSD$_1$ is expressed predominantly in the liver, kidney, testis, and lung. In contrast, 11β-HSD Type 2 (11β-HSD$_2$), also called the kidney isoform, has a K_m below 100 nM. It requires NAD as a cofactor and is predominantly oxidative. In the rat, the adrenal gland, kidney, and distal colon contain the highest amounts of 11β-HSD$_2$. There is further evidence in the literature for the presence of other proteins with 11β-HSD activity; monospecific polyclonal antibodies generated against the 34 kDa liver isoform have revealed several immunologically related forms by Western blot analysis. Two bands were detected in the liver while three bands were detected in the kidney [2]. The specificity of 11β-HSD for hydrocortisone has been analyzed by assessing the ability of other endogenous steroids to interfere with the metabolism of hydrocortisone by 11β-HSD. In general, these studies determined that 11-hydroxy progestins and 11-hydroxy pregnenolone are the most potent inhibitors. Northern blot analyses indicate they do not affect 11β-HSD gene expression.

The activity of both isoforms is influenced by a number of additional factors. Carbenoxolone, the succinic acid derivative of glycyrrhetinic acid, is also a potent 11β-HSD inhibitor (Fig. 2). These compounds differ slightly in their effects, however, in that glycyrrhetinic acid inhibits predominantly the oxidative reaction whereas carbenoxolone inhibits both oxidation and reduction. Moreover, limited studies also suggest that 11β-HSD activity is affected by the presence or absence of endogenous sex steroids. Hepatic 11β-HSD has been

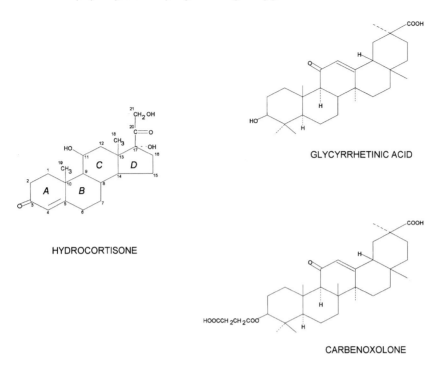

Figure 2. Structure of hydrocortisone and the licorice-derived 11β-HSD inhibitors, glycyrrhetinic acid and carbenoxolone.

shown to be androgen sensitive; enzyme activity is 20-fold higher in the liver and 50% higher in the kidney in male rats compared to females [3]. The pituitary appears to play an important role in this phenomenon, since hypophysectomy increases activity in the female to levels equivalent to those in the male, and the exogenous administration of estradiol decreases activity only in the presence of an intact pituitary.

No x-ray crystallographic studies have been performed for the structural analysis of either 11β-HSD isoform. However, sequence analyses, mutagenesis studies, computer modeling and comparisons to the established structures of related oxidoreductases have provided valuable information as to their probable structures [4]. The amino acid sequences of 11β-HSD$_1$ and 11β-HSD$_2$ are only 28% homologous, yet their tertiary structures are believed to be remarkably similar. Both proteins possess α-helices with an outer hydrophobic surface and are therefore thought to be active as dimers – a property similar to many alcohol dehydrogenases. Furthermore, each monomer possesses a single coenzyme binding domain, located near the amino terminus, which is specific for the cofactors NAD(H) or NADP(H), as well as a single substrate binding domain. These observations put to rest earlier notions that the oxidative and reductive reactions may be conducted by different proteins.

Evidence for regulation of glucocorticoid activity by 11β-HSD

Although both 11β-HSD isoforms are present to some extent in most organs, each isoenzyme is only expressed by a small number of cell types. Furthermore, a given cell type, in general, expresses only one isoform. The presence of multiple forms of the 11β-HSD protein appears to play a pivotal role in the tissue-specific physiologic processes of the organs that produce them (Fig. 3). 11β-HSD$_2$, for instance, is preferentially expressed in organs, such as the kidney and colon, that regulate fluid and electrolytes and possess the type I, or mineralocorticoid, receptor. In contrast, organs that predominantly express the 11β-HSD$_1$ enzyme are most susceptible to the glucocorticoid properties of hydrocortisone. The remainder of this chapter will consider the implications of 11β-HSD activity in the tissues that express these enzymes as well as the potential consequences of pharmacologic alterations in 11β-HSD activity.

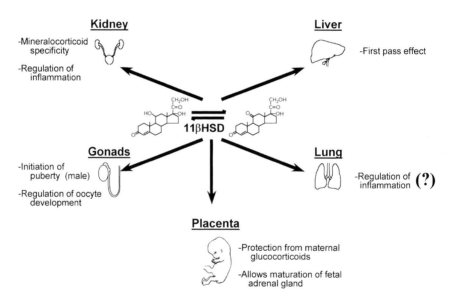

Figure 3. Organs in which 11β-HSD activity has been detected. Listed for each organ are the tissue-specific functions in which 11β-HSD has been implicated.

Regulation of the effects of steroids on renal function by 11β-HSD

In vitro studies have shown that hydrocortisone has approximately equal affinity for the mineralocorticoid receptor as aldosterone. However, aldosterone, with circulating levels that are approximately 1000-fold lower, is the primary regulator of sodium uptake. This apparent paradox was resolved by the findings of Funder et al. who suggested a mechanism by which 11β-HSD regulates the mineralocorticoid responses of the kidney [5]. He proposed that in the kidney, 11β-HSD transforms hydrocortisone locally to its inactive metabolite cortisone, leaving aldosterone free to bind the mineralocorticoid receptor unimpeded (Fig. 4). This was supported and extended by the observation that hydrocortisone is converted to cortisone in the kidney, parotid, and colon – organs that possess both the mineralocorticoid receptor and mineralocorticoid activity. Organs that possess the mineralocorticoid receptor but do not manifest

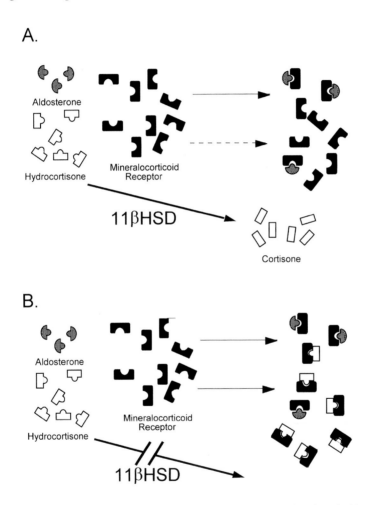

Figure 4. Renal 11β-HSD prevents binding of hydrocortisone to the mineralocorticoid receptor. Although both hydrocortisone and aldosterone bind the mineralocorticoid receptor with equal affinities *in vitro*, hydrocortisone is converted to the inactive glucocorticoid cortisone, leaving aldosterone as the sole regulator of mineralocorticoid activity (A). When 11β-HSD is congenitally absent, as in the syndrome of Apparent Mineralocorticoid Excess, or pharmacologically inhibited, as by the licorice-derived compound glycyrrhetinic acid, both hydrocortisone and aldosterone bind the mineralocorticoid receptor, resulting in excessive mineralocorticoid activation (B).

11β-HSD activity, such as the hippocampus and heart, are not known to actively regulate salt or fluid balance.

The relevance of 11β-HSD to mineralocorticoid activity is further supported by the development of salt retention, hypertension, and edema in patients who are treated with high doses of carbenoxolone or in those who consume excessive amounts of licorice (which contains inhibitors to 11β-HSD; see above). Furthermore, 11β-HSD$_2$ has now been localized to the ascending loop of Henle and collecting duct where aldosterone is known to exert its effects [2]. The congenital deficiency of 11β-HSD$_2$ results in the syndrome of Apparent Mineralocorticoid Excess (AME). Patients with this syndrome suffer from excessive activation of the mineralocorticoid receptors, despite normal to low levels of all mineralocorticoid hormones, resulting in severe hypertension, edema, and hypokalemia. Failure to convert hydrocortisone to cortisone results in elevated urinary excretion of the 11β-hydroxy metabolites of hydrocortisone (tetrahydrocortisol and C-19 steroids) and reduced excretion of the 11-oxo metabolites (cortolones and tetrahydrocortisone). Treatment consists of the administration of dexamethasone which does not activate the mineralocorticoid receptor but suppresses the hypothalamic-pituitary-adrenal axis, thereby minimizing hydrocortisone production.

The kidney is also known to express 11β-HSD$_1$ which has been localized to the proximal nephron and mesangial bed by immunohistochemistry studies. Its proximal location and relatively low affinity for hydrocortisone effectively rules out any significant impact on mineralocorticoid activity. Recent observations show that 11β-HSD$_1$ inhibition in rat mesangial cells potentiates the ability of the rat glucocorticoid corticosterone to suppress secretion of group II phospholipase A2, a key enzyme producing inflammatory mediators [6]. Furthermore, 11β-HSD reductive activity is increased by the inflammatory cytokines TNFα and IL-1β. These findings suggest that renal 11β-HSD$_1$ may modulate the natural course of renal inflammatory disorders, such as glomerulonephritis, by increasing local levels of endogenous glucocorticoids.

Regulation of blood pressure by 11β-HSD-dependent changes in glucocorticoid levels

The effects of glucocorticoids on blood pressure regulation have been recognized for over 50 years. The prevalence of elevated blood pressure among patients with Cushing's disease is approximately 75%. Glucocorticoids also potentiate the sensitivity of vascular smooth muscle cells for catecholamines and have been shown to increase adrenoreceptor number and enhance receptor coupling to stimulatory G-proteins [7]. Finally, glucocorticoids inhibit inducible nitric oxide synthase in vascular smooth muscle cells and the consequent production of the potent vasodilator nitric oxide [8].

11β-HSD$_1$ has been localized to vascular smooth muscle cells and its activity is greatest in resistance vessels (mesenteric and caudal arteries), suggesting it may participate in glucocorticoid-dependent effects on blood pressure. The relevance of 11β-HSD to blood pressure regulation is supported by the finding that licorice ingestion enhances dermal vasoconstriction by hydrocortisone, but not by beclomethasone, a glucocorticoid that is not inactivated by 11β-HSD [9]. That the half-life of 11α-^{3}H-cortisol is prolonged in hypertensive patients relative to controls has been suggested to imply that a dysregulation of 11β-HSD activity may contribute to the development of essential hypertension [10]. In a study of hypertensives, the half-life of 11α-^{3}H-cortisol was distributed in a *bimodal* fashion; 35% of patients demonstrating half-lives greater than two standard deviations above the control means. These patients did not display hypokalemia or reductions in renin or aldosterone; thus, the hypertension was not thought to be related to excessive mineralocorticoid receptor activation.

Placental 11β-HSD activity has also been associated with the development of adult hypertension. The placenta expresses predominantly the 11β-HSD$_2$ isoform whose activity is overwhelmingly oxidative (i.e., hydrocortisone to cortisone). As a result, the fetus is protected from the transmission of maternal glucocorticoids, which circulate at levels five to ten times higher than those in the fetus. Fetal exposure to glucocorticoids is strongly associated with the subsequent development of hypertension in laboratory animals [11]. Interestingly, placental 11β-HSD activity correlates directly with birth weight and inversely with placental weight. Fetuses with low birth weight and high placental weight, which in humans are at the highest risk of subsequent hypertension, had the lowest 11β-HSD activity, and therefore presumably the highest exposure to maternal glucocorticoids. When placental 11β-HSD is inhibited in rats with carbenoxolone, subsequent offspring are significantly more likely to develop hypertension as adults [12]. The mechanisms by which the exposure to glucocorticoids *in utero* may program hypertension later in life are not entirely clear, but may relate to irreversible changes in structure of the vasculature or the central nervous system.

Regulation of ovary and testis function by 11β-HSD

In addition to the pituitary-derived hormones follicle-stimulating hormone (FSH) and luteinizing hormone (LH), adrenal steroids are also believed to suppress gonadal development and gametogenesis. In many mammalian species, for example, reproductive function is suppressed in low-ranking members of a population. This subfertility of social subordinates is often associated with significantly higher levels of circulating cortisol [13]. In humans, elevated circulating glucocorticoids have been associated with the high prevalence of infertility among patients with Cushing's Disease or anorexia nervosa [14].

Glucocorticoids are known to specify the expression of gonadotropic hormones in the hypothalamus and anterior pituitary. However, the observation that glucocorticoid receptors exist on ovarian and testicular cells as well as the finding that glucocorticoids directly affect gonadal steroidogenesis *in vitro* suggest that local effects are also important. Whereas glucocorticoids have a predominantly inhibitory effect on steroid production by testis Leydig cells, their effect on ovarian cells varies with the ovarian cycle. In rat and human granulosa cells that have not undergone luteinization, glucocorticoids stimulate the activity of the steroid-producing enzymes aromatase and 17β-HSD. In contrast, in granulosa-lutein cells (i.e., after luteinization) glucocorticoids have an *inhibitory* effect on progesterone release [15].

11β-HSD activity was first demonstrated in the human ovary by Murphy and has subsequently also been found in the testis [16]. In the ovary, both 11β-HSD mRNA and enzyme activity have been localized to the granulosa-lutein cells. In contrast, 11β-HSD has not been found in the granulosa cells of the pre-ovulatory follicle. Although there is presently no data demonstrating a direct role for 11β-HSD in the ovary, its function in this organ has been open to some debate. Michael has hypothesized that 11β-HSD serves as a temporal regulator of glucocorticoid activity in the ovary [17]; 11β-HSD activity is suppressed during the follicular phase of the ovarian cycle when glucocorticoids are necessary for oocyte maturation. However, during the luteal phase when circulating glucocorticoids would inhibit LH-dependent progesterone biosynthesis, 11β-HSD activity is present.

The relevance of 11β-HSD to ovarian function is further supported by the observation that in women undergoing *in-vitro* fertilization and embryo transfer (IVF-ET), the presence of 11β-HSD activity in cultured granulosa-lutein cells is associated with an unsuccessful outcome. Of 64 patients studied that underwent IVF-ET in a British study, none of the 32 women who had detectable 11β-HSD activity became pregnant [18]. Of the remaining patients without evidence of 11β-HSD activity, 76% achieved successful pregnancies. These findings are consistent with those stated earlier, i.e., that a high cortisol/low 11β-HSD environment is necessary for successful oocyte development. The presence of detectable 11β-HSD activity in cultured cells of unsuccessful IVF-ET procedures may reflect premature functional luteinization of the ovarian follicle prior to oocyte retrieval. Also of note, successful outcomes were not accompanied by improved rates of fertilization, but rather by higher rates of implantation. This suggests that the absence of 11β-HSD activity may allow improved survival of the fetal allograft due to the immunosuppressive properties of glucocorticoids.

In the Leydig cells of the testis, the relative activity of 11β-HSD$_1$ is two to three times that of the liver and the highest of any cell type. Circumstantial evidence suggests that this enzyme may regulate the suppressive effects of glucocorticoids on Leydig cell testosterone secretion. 11β-HSD expression is suppressed in the pre-pubescent testis; its presence coincides with the initiation of testicular testosterone secretion [19]. That these observations are due to direct effects of glucocorticoids in the absence of involvement by the pituitary or hypothalamus is supported by the finding that glucocorticoids suppress testosterone secretion by Leydig cells in culture.

Role of 11β-HSD on lung development and function

Glucocorticoids have been associated with a variety of functions in the fetal and adult lung. In the fetus, glucocorticoids are necessary for the initiation and maintenance of surfactant synthesis prior to birth. In the adult, glucocorticoids are potent inhibitors of inflammation and are used commercially in the treatment of inflammatory disorders, such as asthma. This section will review the importance of glucocorticoids in the fetal and adult lung, as well as how glucocorticoid function in the lung may be modulated by 11β-HSD.

The role of 11β-HSD in the development of the fetal lung
A number of physiologic changes occur prior to birth to enhance glucocorticoid activity. Adrenal glucocorticoid secretion, relatively low in early gestation, increases steadily. Furthermore, levels of glucocorticoid receptors in the lung rise just prior to birth. Premature birth increases the risk of developing the respiratory distress syndrome (RDS), a life-threatening disorder in which immature alveolar Type II cells do not secrete sufficient quantities of surfactant to prevent alveolar collapse. Although patients with this condition possess lower levels of circulating glucocorticoid relative to control, this difference decreases as their delivery approach full-term. The importance of glucocorticoids to the pathogenesis of this disorder is further supported by the findings that hydrocortisone increases synthesis of the surfactant component lecithin in fetal lung cells *in vitro* and that the administration of glucocorticoids to mothers in premature labor significantly decreases the incidence and morbidity of RDS [20]. 11β-HSD is expressed in the fetal lung and its activity disappears shortly before birth. The absence of 11β-HSD in late gestation may therefore contribute to the late-gestational rise of fetal glucocorticoid levels.

The effects of 11β-HSD on inflammation in the adult lung
Glucocorticoids have been widely studied in the adult airway and are presently first-line agents in the treatment of inflammatory diseases, such as asthma. That 11β-HSD is physiologically active in the lung is suggested by gas chromatography-mass spectrometry studies in which the hydrocortisone/cortisone ratio in BAL fluid was found to be approximately 10% of that found in plasma, implying that 11β-HSD converts the majority of 11β-HSD in the airways to cortisone [21]. Theoretically, increased 11β-HSD could contribute to inflammatory conditions in the lung by decreasing local levels of active glucocorticoid. While often these conditions result from altered expression of glucocorticoid receptors and/or transcription factors, increased metabolism of hydrocortisone could also contribute to steroid resistance.

Data concerning an important pulmonary role of 11β-HSD have been mixed. 11β-HSD activity in the lung has been localized to epithelial cells lining the airway. Incubation of these cells with the 11β-HSD inhibitor glycyrrhetinic acid potentiates the ability of hydrocortisone to inhibit GM-CSF release by these cells, suggesting that this enzyme may play a role in modu-

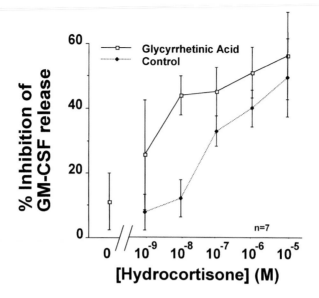

Figure 5. Glycyrrhetinic acid potentiates the inhibition of GM-CSF by hydrocortisone in human primary bronchial epithelial cells (PBEC). PBEC were preincubated with hydrocortisone at the indicated concentrations +/– glycyrrhetinic acid (10^{-6} M). Cells were stimulated with 5 ng/ml IL-1β and GM-CSF levels were quantitated by ELISA. Data shown are the mean+/–SEM percent inhibition of GM-CSF from seven experiments. Incubation with hydrocortisone resulted in a dose-dependent suppression of GM-CSF release (IC_{50}-5.0 $\times$ 10^{-8} M) which was significantly potentiated by coincubation with glycyrrhetinic acid (IC_{50}-1.5 $\times$ 10^{-9} M).

lating inflammatory activity (Fig. 5) [22]. There exists conflicting information, however, concerning whether 11β-HSD activity itself is altered by inflammatory conditions. Lavages of the nasal epithelium, which is phenotypically similar to bronchial epithelium, before and after allergen challenge in allergic subjects result in a slight increase in the hydrocortisone/cortisone ratio (unpublished data). However, 11β-HSD activity, as measured by the relative conversion of [^{3}H]hydrocortisone to [^{3}H]cortisone or [^{3}H]cortisone to [^{3}H]hydrocortisone, is not altered in primary bronchial epithelial cells incubated *in vitro* with the inflammatory cytokines TNFα, IL-1β, IL-4, and IL-8 (unpublished data). Currently, there have been no *in vivo* studies to determine whether 11β-HSD expression is altered in some instances of lung pathologies, and such studies certainly seem warranted.

Therapeutic importance of 11β-HSD manipulation

Several lines of evidence now suggest that endogenous glucocorticoids play a greater role in airway inflammation than previously realized. For instance, after the administration of inhaled allergen, plasma samples from patients who manifest a late asthmatic response contain lower levels of hydrocortisone than those that did not [23]. Animal studies reveal that the administration of metyrapone, an inhibitor of adrenal glucocorticoid synthesis, dramatically potentiates the late asthmatic response in dogs [24]. Theoretically, by potentiating the properties of hydrocortisone, long-term 11β-HSD inhibitors could exert a significant anti-inflammatory effect. Indeed, carbenoxolone, a succinic acid derivative of glycyrrhetinic acid, is currently employed therapeutically in the United Kingdom and other countries as a topical treatment for herpetic stomatitis. Although the systemic use of carbenoxolone, when used as an anti-ulcer medication in the 1960s and 1970s, was associated with salt retention and edema, no such side-effects were seen with topical therapy [25]. Topical treatments could be expanded to inflammatory conditions of the lung where 11β-HSD inhibitors could have a profound glucocorticoid-like effect if administered by inhalation. If effective, they would conceivably allow the dose of synthetic glucocorticoids to be reduced, thereby minimizing the side-effects associated with exogenously administered glucocorticoids. Although more work is clearly needed in this area, the observations discussed herein may open the door for new 11β-HSD-based therapies in the treatment of disease.

Summary

The enzyme 11β-HSD interconverts hydrocortisone, the major active endogenous glucocorticoid in humans, and its inactive metabolite cortisone. Two forms are known to exist: a low affinity isoform, 11β-HSD$_1$, found in glucocorticoid-sensitive tissues, and a high affinity isoform, 11β-HSD$_2$, found in mineralocorticoid-sensitive tissues. The preferential expression of either isoform permits organ-specific regulation of hydrocortisone activity at a local level. In the kidney, 11β-HSD$_2$ prevents hydrocortisone from binding the mineralocorticoid receptor, leaving aldosterone as the sole regulator of mineralocorticoid activity. In gonadal tissue, the temporal regulation of 11β-HSD activity modulates successful oocyte development in females, and the onset of puberty in males. In the lung, 11β-HSD permits successful lung maturation before birth and may modulate airway inflammation in the adult. These findings suggest that 11β-HSD inhibitors may be useful clinically in regulating hydrocortisone action.

References

1 Persson CGA (1989) Glucocorticoids for asthma – early contributions. *Pulmonary Pharmacol* 2: 163–166
2 Monder C, White (PC) (1992) Biochemistry, molecular biology, and physiology of 11β-hydroxysteroid dehydrogenase. *In*: Edward CRW, DW Lincoln (eds): *Recent advances in endocrinology and metabolism*. Churchill Livingstone, Edinburgh, 4: 1–19
3 Lax ER, Ghraf R, Schriefers H (1978) The hormonal regulation of hepatic microsomal 11β-

hydroxysteroid dehydrogenase activity in the rat. *Acta Endocrinol* 89: 267

4 Tsigelny I, Baker ME (1995) Structures important in mammalian 11β and 17β-hydroxysteroid dehydrogenases. *J Steroid Biochem Mol Biol* 55: 589–600

5 Funder JW, Pearce PT, Smith R, Smith AI (1988) Mineralocorticoid action: target tissue specificity is enzyme, not receptor, mediated. *Science* 241: 340–349

6 Escher G, Galli I, Vishwanath BS, Frey BM, Frey FJ (1997) Tumor necrosis factor α and interleukin 1β enhance the cortisone/cortisol shuttle. *J Exp Med* 186: 189–198

7 Haigh RM, Jones CT, Milligan G (1990) Glucocorticoids regulate the amount of G proteins in rat aorta. *J. Mol Endocrinol* 5: 185–188

8 Rees DD, Cellek S, Palmer RMJ, Moncada S (1990) Dexamethasone prevents the induction by endotoxin of a nitric oxide synthase and the associated effects on vascular tone: an insight into endotoxic shock. *Biochem Biophys Res Commun* 173: 541–547

9 Walker BR, Connacher AA, Webb DJ, Edwards CRW (1992) Glucocorticoids and blood pressure: a role for the cortisol/cortisone shuttle in the control of vascular tone in man. *Clin Sci* 83: 171–178

10 Walker BR Stewart PM, Shackleton CHL, Padfield PL, Edwards CRW (1993) Deficient inactivation of cortisol by 11β-hydroxysteroid dehydrogenase in essential hypertension. *Clin Endocrinol* 39: 221–227

11 Benediktsson R, Lindsay RS, Noble J, Seckl JR, Edwards CRW (1993) Glucocorticoid exposure *in utero*: a new model for adult hypertension. *Lancet* 341: 339–341

12 Lindsay RS, Lindsay RM, Edwards CRW, Seckl JR (1996) Inhibition of 11β-hydroxysteroid dehydrogenase in pregnant rats and the programming of blood pressure in the offspring. *Hypertension* 27: 1200–1204

13 Sapolsky R (1985) Stress-induced suppression of testicular function in the wild baboon: role of glucocorticoids. *Endocrinology* 116: 2273–2278

14 Schweiger U, Pirke KM, Laessle RG, Fitcher MM (1992) Gonadotropin secretion in bulimia nervosa. *J Clin Endocrinol Metab* 74: 1122–1127

15 Fateh M, Ben-Rafael Z, Benadiva CA, MastroianniL, Flickinger GL (1989) Cortisol levels in human follicular fluid. *Fertil Steril* 51: 538–541

16 Murphy BE (1981) Ontogeny of cortisol-cortisone interconversion in human tissues: a role for cortisone in human fetal development. *J Steroid Biochem* 14: 811–817

17 Michael AE, Cooke BA (1994) A working hypothesis for the regulation of steroidogenesis and germ cell development in the gonads by glucocorticoids and 11β-hydroxysteroid dehydrogenase. *Mol Cell Endocrinol* 100: 55–63

18 Michael AE, Gregory L, Walker SM, Antoniw JW, Shaw RW, Edwards CRW, Cooke BA (1993) Ovarian 11β-hydroxysterid dehydrogenase: potential predictor of conception by *in vitro* fertilisation and embryo transfer. *Lancet* 342: 711–712

19 Phillips DM, Lakshmi V, Monder C (1989) Corticosteroid 11β-dehydrogenase in rat testis. *Endocrinology* 125: 209–216

20 Liggins GC, Howie RN (1972) A controlled trial of antepartum glucocorticoid treatment for prevention of the respiratory distress syndrome in premature infants. *Pediatrics* 50: 515–525

21 Hubbard WC, Bickel C, Schleimer RP (1994) Simultaneous quantitation of endogenous levels of cortisone and cortisol in human nasal and bronchoalveolar lavage fluids and plasma *via* gas chromatography-negative ion chemical ionization mass spectrometry. *Anal Biochem* 221: 109–117

22 Feinstein MB, Schleimer RP (1999) Regulation of the action of hydrocortisone in airway epithelial cells by 11β-hydroxysteroid dehydrogenase. *Amer J Respir Cell Mol Biol* 21: 403–408

23 Peebles RS, Bickel C, Brennan F, Hubbard W, Togias A, Schleimer RP (1996) Measurement of endogenous glucocorticoids in patients with asthma and in healthy subjects: relationship to allergen-induced changes in lung function. *Amer J Respir Crit Care Med* 153:A879

24 Sasaki H, Yanai M, Shimura S, Okayama H, Aikawa T, Sasaki T, Takishima T (1987) Late asthmatic response to Ascaris antigen challenge in dogs treated with metyrapone. *Amer Rev Respir Dis* 136: 1459–1465

25 Partridge M, Poswillo DE (1984) Topical carbenoxolone sodium in the management of herpes simplex infections. *Brit J Oral Maxillofacial Surg* 22: 138–145

Glucocorticoids in contemporary clinical practice

Glucocorticoids and asthma

John H. Toogood

The London Health Sciences Centre, South Campus (Victoria), Allergy Clinic, 800 Commissioners Road, East, London, Ontario, Canada N6A 4G5

Introduction

Bronchial asthma is primarily a chronic inflammatory disease of the bronchopulmonary airways associated with an intramural infiltration of lymphocytes and eosinophils, and an excess production of T_{H2} type cytokines.

It is characterized by airways hyperresponsiveness, manifested by reversible bronchospasm, and exacerbated by intermittent exposure to respirable irritants or allergens or respiratory infections and, in some individuals, by the ingestion of acetylsalicylic acid or similar nonsteroidal antiinflammatory drugs.

The principle objectives of asthma treatment are to identify and avoid the causative factors and to control the primary airways inflammation with medication. Among the anti-inflammatory medications currently available to treat asthma, the glucocorticoids are the most effective. A stepwise approach to its pharmacologic therapy is advocated, based on the clinical severity of the disease: mild intermittent, mild persistent, moderate persistent, or severe persistent [1].

Mechanisms of glucocorticoid action

The important antiinflammatory effects of glucocorticoids (GC) in the bronchopulmonary airways include inhibition of the production of T_{H2}-type lymphocyte cytokines and pro-inflammatory mediators; inhibition of leucocyte priming or activation; decreases in vascular permeability; inhibition of the release of arachidonic acid metabolites and platelet-activating factor; synergistic or permissive effects on cell responsiveness to other hormones such as catecholamines; and modulation of the overall process by inhibition of the synthesis or release of a variety of inflammatory enzymes, and by induction of the synthesis of other enzymes that have direct antiinflammatory properties.

This exceptionally broad spectrum of activities allows GC to interfere with the primary pathogenetic process of asthma at many different points. In contrast, the antiinflammatory action of other nonsteroidal classes of antiasthmatic drugs, such as the antileukotrienes, is much more narrowly focused and their therapeutic potential is, in consequence, more limited.

Inhaled formulations of glucocorticoid (IGC) are inherently more efficient than oral or parenteral GC, because the ratio of their antiasthmatic to systemic potencies is much more favourable. At low doses, the clinical efficacy of IGC appears fully explainable by their topical actions in the airways. The bioactive fraction that is systemically absorbed appears neither essential for, nor contributory to, their therapeutic activity [2]. At high doses, the possibility of a supererogatory effect from systemically absorbed drug cannot be excluded. In light of these pharmacologic and clinical properties, IGCs now occupy a pivotal position in the treatment of chronic asthma.

Inhaled glucocorticoids: efficacy

Clinical benefits

IGC treatment has been shown to reduce all aspects of asthma morbidity [3] and the associated health care costs. It has proven to be more effective than alternative nonsteroidal antiinflammatory asthma drugs such as cromoglycate or nedocromil [3] and to be associated with lower asthma mortality than that of patients with severe asthma treated with bronchodilators alone or bronchodilators plus cromoglycate [4].

These favourable outcomes reflect the capacity of IGC to improve pulmonary impairment and the accompanying airways hyperresponsiveness. Some aspects of the hyperresponsiveness begin to respond within 6 h of commencing the therapy, but months or years of regular treatment may be required to achieve a maximal response. Even so, few patients achieve a fully normal value [5] (Fig. 1). Symptom and airflow indices respond more quickly, typically within days or weeks.

In addition to its normalizing effect on asthmatic pulmonary impairment, several long-term controlled studies indicate that IGCs at low or high dosage may attenuate or possibly prevent the progression of variable functional impairment to non-reversible chronic airflow limitation. Furthermore, the earlier in the clinical course of the asthma that IGC therapy is started, the more effective it appears to be in this regard [6].

Determinants of efficacy

The dose per day, drug delivery system, duration of therapy and the management system used to ensure good patient compliance with the prescribed treatment are major determinants of the success or failure of IGC therapy.

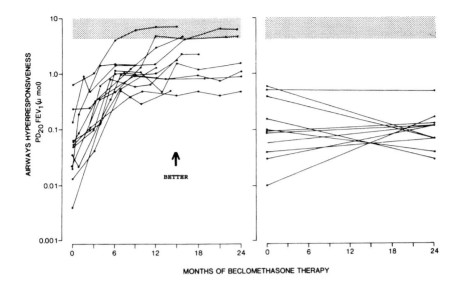

Figure 1. Left: Shows the gradual improvement of airways hyperresponsiveness in response to low-dose beclomethasone in a group of patients who participated in a structured treatment plan that included daily recording of PEF. Values for PD_{20} in the shaded zone above 4.0 are normal. The patients on the right, who received the same drug without a structured plan for therapy, failed to improve their airways hyperresponsiveness despite 2 years of treatment. The results of inhaled steroid therapy are critically dependent on the clinical management system used by the physician to ensure good patient compliance. (Adapted from [5].)

Daily dosage

The benefits and adverse effects of IGC are dose dependent [7, 8] with the ED_{50} or the "toxic" dose being determined by which response index is chosen to measure the drug's effect. In general, symptoms tend to respond at a lower dose than measures of functional impairment [3]. Patients vary widely in respect to their minimum maintenance dose requirements during long-term treatment (Tab. 1). These dose requirements provide an empirical basis for categorizing different levels of chronic asthma severity.

As recommended in current guidelines [1, 9], it is advantageous to begin a trial of IGC with a high rather than a low dose. If the daily dose is too low in patients with moderate to severe asthma, the therapeutic response may be slow, and it may plateau and persist at a level well short of normal. Suboptimal IGC treatment is reportedly common among both adults and children [6].

Tachyphylaxis has not been observed in patients treated initially with high doses. On the contrary, the daily dose of IGC may be successfully down-titrated over a period of months or years while maintaining the benefits secured with the initial high dosage [6]. As the inflammatory process subsides, the binding affinity of the GC receptor increases. Furthermore, the down-regula-

Table 1. Frequency distribution of daily doses of budesonide or beclomethasone required in clinical practice[*]

Daily dose (mg)[†]	Number of patients using I-S	Percent of I-S users (n = 296)	Cumulative percent (n = 296)
0.01	1	0.34	0.34
0.02	1	0.34	0.68
0.03	1	0.34	1.01
0.05	2	0.68	1.69
0.10	2	0.68	2.36
0.17	1	0.34	2.70
0.20	19	6.42	9.12
0.25	1	0.34	9.46
0.30	12	4.05	13.51
0.36	1	0.34	13.85
0.40	37	12.50	26.35
0.50	7	2.36	28.72
0.60	11	3.72	32.43
0.62	1	0.34	32.77
0.65	1	0.34	33.11
0.68	1	0.34	33.45
0.75	5	1.69	35.14
0.80	56	18.92	54.39
0.90	1	0.34	54.73
1.00	33	11.15	65.88
1.02	1	0.34	66.22
1.08	1	0.34	66.55
1.10	1	0.34	66.89
1.20	27	9.12	76.01
1.30	1	0.34	76.35
1.37	1	0.34	76.69
1.50	8	2.70	79.39
1.54	1	0.34	79.73
1.60	31	10.47	90.20
1.76	1	0.34	90.54
1.80	5	1.69	92.23
2.00	8	2.70	94.93
2.06	1	0.34	95.27
2.25	1	0.34	95.61
2.40	7	2.36	97.97
2.50	1	0.34	98.31
3.20	5	1.69	100.00

[*] Utilization data from a 1989–90 audit of all adult asthmatic patients receiving ambulatory care from three specialist physicians in a tertiary health care facility (n = 398).
[†] Nominal dose prescribed, corrected for patient-reported dose omissions.
From *Clin Invest Med* (1991) 14(4): A6.

tion of GC receptors initially induced by high dose therapy reverts toward pre-treatment values as the dose is reduced. Both these changes would tend to potentiate the pharmacologic activity of IGC and thus reduce dose require-ments over time.

Drug delivery system

Many patients coordinate their inspiratory effort with the pressurized metered dose inhaler (pMDI) so poorly as to jeopardize the effectiveness of the treat-ment. Instructing the patient in the correct inhalation technique can materially improve drug delivery to the lung, and further improvement can be achieved by attaching a "spacer" device to the pMDI.

Spacers reduce particle velocity and allow more of the propellant to evapo-rate by increasing the transit distance of the aerosol jet. This increases the pro-portion of small particles in the "respirable fraction" capable of accessing the lower airways. Particles deposited in the oropharynx or larger airways serve no useful purpose and may cause oropharyngeal complications or reflex cough or bronchospasm. Efficient usage of a spacer requires that the patient be aware of the many factors that may act to reduce drug delivery through the device. These include (1) failure to shake the pMDI between each puff, which can materially reduce the amount of drug expelled from the canister into the spac-er; (2) variations in the amount of electrostatic charge within the spacer, which act to trap a proportion of the aerosolized drug on its inner surfaces; (3) the dis-charge of more than one puff at a time into the spacer before inhaling the drug; (4) variations in the time-lapse between expelling the drug into the spacer and the start of inspiration; (5) the point in the respiratory cycle at which inspira-tion commences: residual volume or functional residual capacity; (6) the rate at which the drug is inspired; and (7) the presence and duration of a post-inspi-ratory breathhold.

Since most of the systemic activity of the more rapidly metabolized IGC drugs such as fluticasone or budesonide reflects the fraction absorbed from the lung, spacers have the potential to induce parallel changes in the drug's intra-pulmonary delivery and systemic availability.

Newer formulations

One alternative to the conventional hand-activated pMDI is the breath-activat-ed pMDI, designed to automatically release each dose from the canister early in inspiration. This device cannot enhance the results normally achieved in patients who already use, or can be trained to use, their hand-activated pMDI efficiently [10]. However, it may significantly improve intrapulmonary drug delivery in patients who fail to master the conventional pMDI, despite careful instruction [10].

Although the pMDI remains the most widely used delivery device for asthma therapy, non-pressurized, dry-powder formulations appear likely to largely displace the pressurized aerosols in future. One such device, the Turbuhaler increases drug deposition in the lung as much as two-fold in comparison to the pMDI alone [11]. Therefore an appropriate adjustment in daily dosage is indicated when converting from the pMDI without spacer to the dry powder Turbuhaler.

Duration of treatment and compliance

A year or more of treatment may be required to achieve an optimal response to IGCs (Fig. 1) [5]. During this time the clinical management system used to foster good patient compliance may be critically important to the success or failure of the treatment as illustrated in Figure 1.

It is doubtful IGC treatment ever "cures" the disease. Abrupt withdrawal of the drug typically evokes asthma recurrence in most patients, commonly within a month. Longer remissions may be associated with milder disease, longer treatment or higher daily doses. Therefore, once started, the need for regular IGC is likely to continue indefinitely.

In light of this prospect, the risks of IGC treatment need to be considered along with its potential benefits.

Inhaled glucocorticoids: safety

Overview

IGC therapy carries less risk of complicating morbidity and mortality - drug or disease related – than that associated with other antiasthmatic drugs such as prednisone, theophylline or β_2-agonist bronchodilators. Although the risk increases with the daily dose of IGC, serious side-effects are uncommon. Yet many patients harbour sufficient concern about the potential risks of IGCs that it reduces their willingness to use these agents and, in consequence, impairs the quality of the therapeutic response that one is able to achieve in ordinary clinical practice.

These concerns focus mainly on the effects of IGCs on the hypothalamic-pituitary-adrenal (HPA) axis, the eye, on growth in children, and on bone metabolism in adults or children.

HPA axis

Suppression of the HPA axis by IGC is dose-dependent, variable among patients and among different IGC drugs, and smaller in magnitude than that associated with therapeutically equivalent doses of oral glucocorticoids (OGCs) [7, 12].

Although, abnormal test values for HPA function may occur with medium or high doses of IGC and sometimes with low doses, clinically important complications are rare, as judged by the paucity of reported cases. Nevertheless, it is recommended that patients using high dose IGC receive a systemic GC supplement if put at risk of Addisonian crisis in the event of major surgery or trauma or severe metabolic stress.

Ocular effects

Cataracts occur much less commonly with IGC than with oral or parenteral GC therapy [12]. However, the risk exists, increases with the daily and cumulative doses of IGC, may impair vision, and may require corrective surgery. Routine ophthalmologic monitoring for cataract has not been shown to alter its surgical management or outcome.

Primary, open-angle glaucoma may be exacerbated by IGCs [12]. The degree of risk increases with higher daily dosages, but not with the cumulative dose or concomitant intranasal steroid use. Untreated glaucoma carries a risk of irreversible vision impairment. It is therefore prudent to measure intraocular pressure when commencing IGC therapy in patients with a personal or family history of glaucoma, and to monitor it subsequently.

Growth suppression

Growth suppression in children treated with IGC relates to the inhibitory effect of GC on the metabolic turnover of Types I and III collagen [12]. The growth inhibition is dose-dependent, and varies among different IGC drugs and different patients. It is therefore recommended that growth be monitored routinely in all children receiving IGC, regardless of dosage.

There are very few data to document the impact of IGC on the height children ultimately attain at adulthood. The existing data are reassuring. However, it remains possible that the level of risk may be affected adversely by current trends towards the use of larger daily doses, more potent drugs, more efficient delivery systems and/or the use of repetitive bursts of high dose IGC to treat asthma exacerbations

Bone formation

Bone formation may be inhibited and resorption increased by either OGC or IGC [12]. In general, these effects on bone turnover are much less with IGCs than with therapeutically equivalent doses of OGCs. Beclomethasone affects bone metabolism more than therapeutically equivalent or milligram equivalent doses of fluticasone or budesonide, respectively.

Although high doses of IGC may reduce bone density (Fig. 2) [13], there is no firm evidence that this occurs with the low or medium doses most commonly used by children or adults [12]. Fracture prevalence is far higher with OGCs. The very few published reports of fracture complicating IGC therapy involved the administration of high dose beclomethasone to adults in whom co-existing non-steroidal risk factors for osteoporosis were present and untreated. An additive effect of the IGC cannot be excluded in these patients, and appears likely [12].

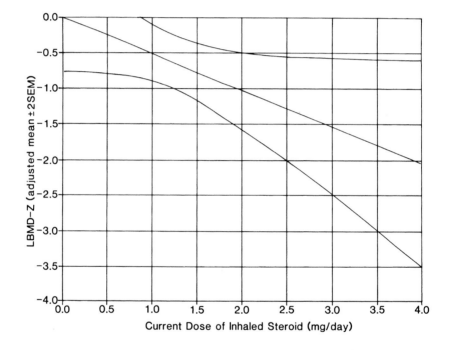

Figure 2. Regression of lumbar spine bone mineral density Z score (LBMD-Z) on the daily dose of inhaled steroid. Dose range: 0–3.2 mg/d of budesonide or beclomethasone. n = 69. Means shown were adjusted by ANCOVA to control for the effects of age, sex, years of estrogen use, physical activity, the current daily dose of prednisone, years of prednisone usage, and the cumulative lifetime dose of inhaled steroid. LBMD-Z declined significantly on the daily dose of inhaled steroid (p = 0.013) [13].

Determinants of risk

All of the antiasthmatic effect and most of the systemic activity of IGC reflects the fraction of each dose delivered to the lung. Therefore increases (or decreases) in the "respirable fraction" of drug and/or the efficiency of the drug delivery system inevitably increase (or decrease) the antiasthmatic and systemic effects of the drug in tandem.

Drug delivery

Different delivery systems may exert major effects on the intrapulmonary and oral delivery of IGC. For example, the Turbuhaler is capable of doubling the intrapulmonary delivery of budesonide in comparison with the pMDI alone. In addition, the patient's inhalation technique may alter the intrapulmonary delivery and systemic availability of the drug by a factor of two or more.

The anticipated changeover from CFC to HFA propellants will require patients using the beclomethasone pressurized aerosol to reduce their daily dose by about 50 to 60%, because the physical properties of the HFA aerosol increase the fraction of each dose which is delivered to the lung and systemically available.

Daily dose

With any IGC, the degree of risk is most effectively minimized by ensuring each patient uses the smallest daily dose sufficient to maintain optimum control of their disease.

Adjunct drugs

In patients who have severe asthma requiring high dose IGC, co-treatment with a "steroid sparing" adjunct along with low or medium dose IGC, can provide an efficacious alternative to increasing the dose of IGC to higher levels. Salmeterol or formoterol are currently recommended for this purpose [1, 9]. The long-term outcome of such treatment remains to be determined. Of concern is the observation that, in persons with atopic asthma, inhaled salbutamol or salmeterol [14] augment the airways smooth muscle and mast cell responses to inhaled allergen or methacholine. These effects cannot be prevented by concurrent inhaled steroid treatment [15]. Thus they might lead, over time, to irreversible fibrosis and smooth muscle hyperplasia causing chronic airflow limitation. These findings favour a conservative approach to the use of a long-acting beta-agonist as a "steroid-sparing" adjunct to IGC, particularly in atopic subjects.

Low dose oral theophylline may be similarly effective as an adjunct, but it carries the potential for inadvertent systemic toxicity. The usefulness of cromoglycate or nedocromil for this purpose is equivocal at best. The value of the new anti-leukotriene agents remains to be established.

Oral or parenteral glucocorticoids for acute asthma

Emergency room or hospital treatment

Placebo-controlled trials clearly demonstrate the efficacy of GC therapy for acute severe asthma [16]. A ventilatory response may be discernible within a few hours in patients previously refractory to beta-agonist bronchodilator therapy because of down-regulation of adrenoreceptors. However at least 5–9 h are required to express the full complement of the antiasthmatic activities of GC. The clinical response then evolves over several days or weeks.

Current guidelines recommend that all patients requiring emergency treatment for severe asthma be considered candidates for oral or intravenous GC therapy – to be administered as soon as possible after initiating inhaled bronchodilator therapy [1, 9, 17].

Oral or parenteral

The oral or intravenous routes of administration do not differ materially in respect to the onset of their clinical effects. Prednisolone bioavailability is approximately equivalent by either route, and oral dosing achieves peak blood levels in an hour or less. Either prednisone or prednisolone may be used since they are rapidly inter-convertible, and the peak levels achieved are influenced more by between-patient differences in the conversion ratio than by which drug was administered. Intravenous therapy may be reserved for patients who are intubated or vomiting or have impaired gastrointestinal absorption.

Dosage

In the emergency room or hospital, the doses of prednisone, prednisolone or methylprednisolone currently recommended for the initial treatment of adults with severe asthma are 120–180 mg/day (USA) [1] or 100–120 mg/day (Canada) [17] – given in three or four divided doses. After 48 h this is normally reduced to 60–80 mg/day (USA) or 30–60 mg/day (Canada), then continued for 3–10 days (USA) or 7–14 days (Canada). This period may vary, depending on the time required to restore the patient's peak expiratory flow (PEF) or forced expiratory volume in one second ($FEV_{1.0}$) to values at least 70% of predicted normal, or to a value previously documented as the maximum attainable by the particular patient. Smaller initial doses of prednisone are recommended in British guidelines: 30–60 mg/d supplemented in selected patients with intravenous hydrocortisone 200 mg [9].

When the OGC is withdrawn, it should immediately be replaced with an IGC [1, 9, 17]. The recommended daily dose of IGC is individualized to each patient and depends on the number of risk-factors present for hospital read-mission or asthma mortality.

Ambulatory care

For the outpatient treatment of moderate to severe exacerbations of asthma, a 3- to 10-day course of prednisone is recommended at a dose of 40–60 mg/day given as a single or two divided doses [1]. Milder exacerbations may be effec-tively treated without OGC by doubling or quadrupling the daily dose of IGC [9, 18]. This is given in four divided doses until the deterioration in PEF has been fully reversed [18].

Oral glucocorticoids for chronic asthma

Inhaled GC therapy is generally conceded to be the treatment of choice for all but the mildest grade of chronic asthma [1]. However, prednisone may be preferable in some circumstances – for example in selected patients in whom adverse socioeconomic circumstances seriously compromise the usefulness of the IGC.

Such patients may need high doses of IGC to achieve and maintain adequate control of their asthma, but cannot be relied upon to take the prescribed dose consistently or to continue it indefinitely. The consequences of failure to com-ply are potentially disastrous as evidenced by their hospitalization and mortal-ity rates. In such high-risk individuals, education may help, provided it is tai-lored to the particular needs and cultural beliefs and priorities of the patient. If all efforts fail, it may be advisable to consider regular prednisone, given alone or in conjunction with a low or intermediate dose of an IGC, rather than rely-ing on IGC alone.

Other conditions requiring continuing OGC therapy include the various forms of systemic necrotizing vasculitis that may be accompanied by asthma [19] and, probably, Allergic Bronchopulmonary Apergillosis (ABPA).

In patients with ABPA, IGC treatment may improve the asthma symptoms without reducing the recurrence rate of segmental pulmonary consolidations. Prednisone, on the other hand, has been shown to prevent these segmental inflammatory lesions. Since it is the destructive effects of the latter rather than the asthma that lead to the widespread lung fibrosis characteristic of end-stage ABPA, OGC therapy should probably remain the mainstay of its long-term management [20]. Opinions vary as to whether patients with mild disease (stage 1 and possibly stage 2) may appropriately be treated with IGC alone. However, the long-term outcome of such treatment has yet to be documented.

Asthma not responsive to glucocorticoids

Typically asthma and exacerbations of asthma are caused by eosinophilic airways inflammation associated with exposure to allergens or occupational chemical sensitizers. However, non-eosinophilic inflammation associated with bacterial or viral infections, smoking, or exposure to endotoxin or ozone may also cause asthma.

Typically the former responds well to GC therapy, but accumulating evidence suggests the latter does not [21]. Research is needed to clarify these associations and their implications with respect to pharmacotherapy.

Summary

Inhaled GC therapy for chronic asthma currently constitutes a *benchmark* of therapeutic efficiency. Therefore the efficiency of new or modified treatment regimens for asthma needs to be established in terms of their clinical performances relative to this benchmark.

References

1 National Asthma Education Program EP (1997) Guidelines for the diagnosis and management of asthma. NIH Publication #97-4051, July 1997. *US Dept of Health and Human Services*, 1–146

2 Toogood JH, Frankish CW, Jennings BH et al (1990) A study of the mechanism of the antiasthmatic action of inhaled budesonide. *J Allergy Clin Immunol* 85: 872–880

3 Toogood JH, Jennings B, Baskerville J, Lefcoe NM (1993) Aerosol corticosteroids. *In*: EB Weiss, M Stein (eds): *Bronchial asthma mechanisms and therapeutics*. Little, Brown and Company, Boston, Mass., 818–841

4 Ernst P, Spitzer WO, Suissa S et al (1992) Risk of fatal and near-fatal asthma in relation to inhaled corticosteroid use. *JAMA* 268: 3462–3464

5 Woolcock AJ, Yan K, Salome CM (1988) Effect of therapy on bronchial hyperresponsiveness in the long-term management of asthma. *Clin Allergy* 18: 165–176

6 Agertoft L, Pedersen S (1994) Effects of long-term treatment with an inhaled corticosteroid on growth and pulmonary function in asthmatic children. *Respir Med* 88: 373–381

7 Toogood JH, Baskerville J, Jennings B, Lefcoe NM, Johansson S (1989) Bioequivalent doses of budesonide and prednisone in moderate and severe asthma. *J Allergy Clin Immunol* 84: 688–700

8 Pauwels RA, Lofdahl C-G, Postma DS et al (1997) Effect of inhaled formoterol and budesonide on exacerbations of asthma. *N Engl J Med* 337: 1405–1410

9 British Thoracic Society (1997) The British guidelines on asthma management. *Thorax* 52: S1–S21

10 Newman SP, Weisz AWB, Talaee N, Clarke SW (1991) Improvement of drug delivery with a breath actuated pressurised aerosol for patients with poor inhaler technique. *Thorax* 46: 712–716

11 Thorsson L, Edsbacker S, Conradson T (1994) Lung deposition of budesonide from turbuhaler is twice that from a pressurized metered-dose inhaler pMDI. *Eur Respir J* 7: 1839–1844

12 Toogood JH (1998) Side-effects of inhaled corticosteroids. *J Allergy Clin Immunol* 102: 705–713

13 Toogood JH, Baskerville JC, Markov AE, Hodsman AB, Fraher LJ, Jennings B, Haddad RG, Drost D (1995) Bone mineral density and the risk of fracture in patients receiving long-term inhaled steroid therapy for asthma. *J Allergy Clin Immunol* 96: 157–166

14 Bhagat R, Kalra S, Swystun VA, Cockcroft DW (1995) Rapid onset of tolerance to the bronchoprotective effect of salmeterol. *Chest* 108: 1235–1239

15 Cockcroft DW, Swystun VA, Bhagat R (1995) Interaction of inhaled B$_2$ agonist and inhaled corticosteroid on airway responsiveness to allergen and methacholine. *Amer J Respir Crit Care Med* 152: 1485–1489

16 Littenberg B, Gluck EH (1986) A controlled trial of methylprednisolone in the emergency treatment of acute asthma. *N Engl J Med* 314: 150–152

17 Beveridge RC, Grunfeld AF, Hodder RV, Verbeek PR (1996) Guidelines for the emergency management of asthma in adults. *Can Med Assn J* 156: 25–37

18 Ernst PM, Fitzgerald JMM, Spier SM (1996) Canadian Asthma Consensus Conference: Summary of Recommendations. *Can Respir J* 3: 89–100

19 Churg A, Brallas M, Cronin SR, Churg J (1995) Formes-frustes of Churg-Strauss syndrome. *Chest* 108: 320–323

20 Greenberger PA (1984) Allergic bronchopulmonary aspergillosis. *J Allergy Clin Immunol* 74: 646–653

21 Pizzichini MMM, Pizzichini E, Clelland L, Efthimiadis A, Mahony J, Dolovich J, Hargreave FE (1997) Sputum in severe exacerbations of asthma: kinetics of inflammatory indices after prednisone treatment. *Amer J Respir Crit Care Med* 155: 1501–1508

Systemic glucocorticoids in chronic arthritis

John R. Kirwan

University Division of Medicine, Bristol Royal Infirmary, Bristol, BS2 8HW, UK

Glucocorticoids offer a mode of treatment for arthritis that has been both seductive and controversial. The history of their use is linked with some of the most important advances in medical science this century. Philip Hench and his colleagues (who were awarded the Nobel Prize for discovering the anti-inflammatory properties of glucocorticoids) used them in rheumatoid arthritis (RA) with dramatic results [1]. The subsequent widespread use of glucocorticoids as anti-inflammatory agents made its mark in many conditions, with an inflammatory or auto-immune basis.

This chapter will review current evidence and practice in the use of glucocorticoids in chronic inflammatory arthritis (typified by RA), in vasculitic episodes typified by those in systemic lupus erythematosus (SLE), and in polymyalgia rheumatica (PMR) and temporal arteritis (TA).

Rheumatoid arthritis and its treatment

Rheumatoid arthritis (RA) is a systemic inflammatory disease that occurs most frequently in the fourth and fifth decades of life and affects primarily the synovial joints. It is chronic and variable, results in considerable morbidity, is associated with an increase in mortality, and is currently incurable. The prevalence of RA in Europe ranges from 1–3% [2]. In the south west of England, patients with RA make up 25% of all new hospital referrals to the Rheumatology clinics and 75% of follow-up work [3].

The management of RA concentrates on the control of joint inflammation, which is seen to be the cause of the immediate day-to-day symptoms and of the gradually accumulating long-term joint damage that occurs in the majority of hospital patients with RA. Non-steroidal anti-infammatory drugs provide the first line of treatment, but a second line of treatment is also able to reduce signs of joint inflammation. Second line agents (also called specific or slow acting anti-rheumatoid drugs) take weeks or months to exert their effect and their mechanism(s) of action are unknown. Currently intramuscular gold (usually sodium aurothiomalate), sulphasalazine, low dose methotrexate, D-penicillamine, cyclosporin A and hydroxy chloroquine are used for this purpose. In severe disease, immunosupressants such as azathioprine and cyclophosphamide may also be used. At the time of writing, new agents designed to work directly on immune system functional mechanisms (such as anti-TNF antibodies) are being introduced, but their role in clinical practice is not yet established.

Much debate has focused on whether or not it is possible to modify sufficiently the natural history of RA to make a difference to long-term patient outcome [4, 5]. This is a difficult question to answer because of the chronic nature of RA and the limitations of present instruments to measure its impact. However, the clinical impression is that medical intervention does have a positive effect on RA and improves outcome as measured by clinical, functional and structural change. The key to long-term outcome probably lies in the control of joint destruction, which accumulates over the years and is seen on radiographs as joint erosions. Whether and by how much joint damage can be prevented or reduced by current and newly developed medications is an active debate. Evidence related to this issue is greatest for glucocorticoids and will be reviewed below.

Initial euphoria at the success of glucocorticoid treatment in RA gave way to disillusionment as clinicians and the public became aware of the serious adverse effects that can occur with prolonged use of high doses. In many countries glucocorticoids became relegated to the bottom of the league table of "second line" therapy for rheumatoid arthritis and were often used only as a last resort for symptom control. However, recent recognition of their potential disease modifying ability in improving function and possibly structural damage has led to a renewed interest and resurgence in their use [6–11].

Glucocorticoids in rheumatoid arthritis – reviewing the evidence

The very short-term anti-inflammatory effect of glucocorticoids has recently been reviewed by Saag [12]. It is clear that, over a few weeks, glucocorticoids have stronger anti-inflammatory effects than non-steroidal anti-inflammatory drugs. However, of greater interest in a chronic condition such as RA is the medium- and long-term effects of treatment. Furthermore, the immune dysfunction in RA is diffuse and glucocorticoids have the potential to influence the immune and inflammatory response at various stages. It seems logical that an agent such as glucocorticoid, which has actions further "upstream" in the pathological pathways than do non-steroidal anti-inflammatory drugs, is more likely to prevent structural damage. In addition, recent evidence suggests that patients with RA may have a defect in the regulation of corticosteroid releasing factor (CRF) by the hypothalamus [13, 14]. In active inflammatory RA serum cortisol levels are reduced and the cortisol response during surgical stress is dampened compared with patients who have osteomyelitis, another chronic inflammatory condition [14]. This raises the possibility that alterations in corticosteroid action or control may play a more fundamental role in the development and progress of RA than previously thought.

Although they have been in use since 1948, there have been relatively few randomised, controlled trials of glucocorticoids in RA, particularly in relation to long-term use. In the early 1950s several attempts were made to define their role. The first of these was conducted by the Medical Research Council (MRC) in conjunction with the Nuffield Foundation in Great Britain [15]. In this study, 61 adult and paediatric patients were randomised to receive cortisone (mean dose 80 mg, equivalent to 16 mg prednisolone) or aspirin (mean dose 4.5 g daily) for 1 year. The study end points included clinical and laboratory parameters but radiological progression was not followed. Patients had their treatment reduced in stages at the end of each 3-month period and final assessments were made 1 week after the drug had been discontinued. The results showed that the acute phase response (measured as the ESR) and haemoglobin levels responded better to cortisone. A series of clinical measures including joint tenderness, range of joint movement, grip strength, disease activity and functional capacity showed improvement in both treatment groups. The authors concluded that, although the corticosteroid patients had some early advantage, by the end of the study there was no difference between the treatments. They noted that patients on glucocorticoids experienced significant withdrawal flares.

A study conducted by the Empire Rheumatism Council [16] randomised 100 adult patients to receive cortisone (mean dose 75 mg daily, equivalent to 14 mg prednisolone) or aspirin (mean dose 4 gm daily) for 2 years. On this occasion x-rays of the hands and feet were taken during the second half of the second year and showed a higher erosion score in the aspirin treated patients, although this did not reach statistical significance (Tab. 1). There were no radiographs at entry so that progression during treatment could not be estimated.

A third trial [17] compared prednisolone (a synthetic analogue of cortisone with greater potency) with aspirin in 84 patients of whom seven did not complete the study. The 41 patients receiving prednisolone had a daily mean dose of 12 mg at the end of the first year and 10 mg at the end of the second year. Thirty-six patients received aspirin. Radiographs were obtained of the hands and feet initially and after 1 and 2 years of treatment and radiographic progression was analysed by assessing a variety of rheumatoid changes including erosions. There were lower rates of progression in erosion scores in the prednisolone group (Tab. 2). At the end of the second year eight patients on analgesics had fared badly and were given prednisolone. During the third year,

Table 1. Proportion (%) of x-rays with definite erosions after 2 years of treatment (from [16])

Hands		Feet	
Cortisone (n = 30)	Aspirin (n = 27)	Cortisone (n = 26)	Aspirin (n = 24)
57	73	41	68

Table 2. Proportion (%) of patients showing x-ray progression after different periods of treatment (from [17])

Time	Prednisolone		Aspirin	
	Hands	Feet	Hands	Feet
1 year	17	12	49	44
2 years	41	10	72	71

5/26 (19%) of patients in the analgesic group progressed but only 4/49 (8%) prednisolone treated patients did so [18]. Four years later West [19] was able to follow-up 74 of the original 77 patients in this study and reported that over 7 years only 9/39 (23%) patients who had continued on prednisolone developed new erosions compared with 32/34 (94%) patients who had continued on aspirin alone. Although this longer term follow-up was uncontrolled, most patients had, in fact, continued with their initial therapy and so this evidence appears persuasive. Published in 1967, in a journal not readily accessible and with a title which did not indicate the nature of the findings, this paper went unnoticed until referenced by Masi in 1983 [20].

Meanwhile a variety of short-term inconclusive studies were published which did not satisfactorily address the question of alteration in radiological progression (Tab. 3). Berntsen [21] compared 183 RA patients on either hydrocortisone, cortisone, prednisolone, prednisone, dexamethasone or triamcinolone against patients already on gold (n = 155) or analgesics alone (n = 50). The period of follow-up was at least 5 years. Radiological progression was present in both groups, leading the authors to conclude that glucocorticoids were no better than gold or analgesics, even though functional capacity was well maintained in the glucocorticoid treated group. There are several important weaknesses in this study: the formulations and doses of glucocorticoids varied widely; the control group(s) had not been randomised; and (in keeping with thinking at that time) glucocorticoids would have been used generally in more aggressive disease, certainly in comparison with an analgesic group. Indeed, three-quarters of the patients in the steroid group had previously failed to respond to gold.

Three other randomised trials were published in 1981, 1983 and 1984 [22–24]. The first showed no advantage for monthly intravenous methylprednisolone compared with placebo over a 6-month period. The second was a small study involving only 18 patients. The authors concluded that erosive progression was less in the prednisolone treated group compared with placebo over a 10-month period. The third study compared patients treated with prednisolone (mean dosage 10.3 mg a day) with those without prednisolone. This study included 103 patients followed up over a period of 120 months. The suggestion from this study was that the hand x-rays showed significantly less erosions in the prednisolone treated group. In a later study comparing pulse intra-

Table 3. Some randomised controlled trials of corticosteroids in rheumatoid arthritis

Study	Year	Ref	No of patients	Treatment (mg/day)	Comparator	Duration (months)	Radiographic result	Comments
MRC	1954	15	61	Cortisone 80	Aspirin 4.5 g/d	12	Not assessed	Withdrawal flares
ERC	1955	16	100	Cortisone 69	Aspirin 4 g/d	12	Non significant but higher porosis and erosion scores in aspirin group	Erosion score could have been refined. If cut off taken at moderate to severe scores, cortisone did far better
MRC	1959	17 18	77	Prednisolone 12 for year 1, 10 for year 2.	Aspirin	36	Less after 1 and 2 years	Followed up for 3 years. Prednisolone probably held advantage into third year
Berntsen	1961	21	183	Hydrocortisone 25 – 100	Analgesics, 50 I/M gold	>60	No difference (steroid group had better functional outcome)	Poorly matched, different doses and formulations, steroid group worse at start.
West	1967	19	74	Prednisolone <15	Aspirin	84	Less progression	10 mg better than 7.5 mg Publication not readily accessable
Liebling	1981	27	10	Methylprednisolone 1 g/mth	Placebo	6	No difference	Very few patients
Harris	1983	23	18	Prednisolone 5	Placebo and crossover at 24/52	10	Less progression in steroid group (and better functional outcome)	Very few patients
Million	1984	24	103	Prednisolone 10.3	No steroids	120	Less erosions	Broad treatment comparison with contamination between groups
Hansen	1990	25	97	Methylprednisolone 1 g i/v monthly	iv saline	12	No difference in erosion scores	
ARC	1995	9,10	128	Prednisolone 7.5	Placebo	24	Reduced erosive change	
COBRA	1997	11	155	Prednisolone, methotrexate and sulphasalazine	Sulphasallazine	9, 11	Reduced erosive change	

venous methylprednisolone with saline infusion, no long-term benefit was found in terms of clinical outcome or radiological progression [25].

In 1986, Byron and Kirwan [26] reviewed and re-analysed the results of both the 1959 MRC trial [17] and the follow-up report by West [19], and concluded that there was a good case for the disease modifying potential of corticosteroid therapy. They proposed the conduct of a new randomised, double-blind, placebo controlled trial of glucocorticoids designed specifically to test the hypothesis that glucocorticoids can suppress erosive progression. The results of that study have been published [9, 10]. This multicentre trial recruited 128 patients with RA of less than 2 years since diagnosis and compared placebo treatment with prednisolone 7.5 mg daily. Patients were allowed to continue on routine medication including second line agents. The patients treated with prednisolone had greater reductions than the placebo group in the number of inflamed joints (articular index), pain (Fig. 1a) and disability during the first few months of the treatment, but were indistinguishable from them during the second year of treatment and after withdrawal of glucocorticoid therapy. There was no difference between the groups for standardised scores for the acute phase response.

The development of erosions and radiological progression were assessed by changes in the Larsen score [31]. After 2 years the Larsen score had shown very little change in the prednisolone treated patients while the placebo group had substantial joint destruction (p = 0.004). This effect was lost during the 1-year blinded post-treatment follow-up (Fig. 1b). In addition, there was an effect on preventing the onset of erosions, as well as their progression (Tab. 4). One can conclude from this study that a fixed daily low dose of prednisolone (7.5 mg) can reduce the rate of radiological progression over 2 years in patients with early RA who are taking concomitant treatment with other second line agents.

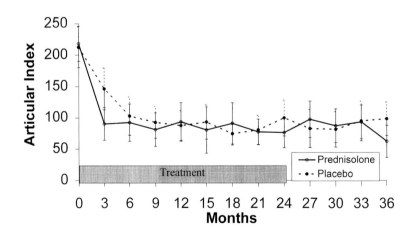

Figure 1a. Mean (95% CI) articular index for 75 patients with radiographs at all time points. The difference between groups is significant at 3 months only.

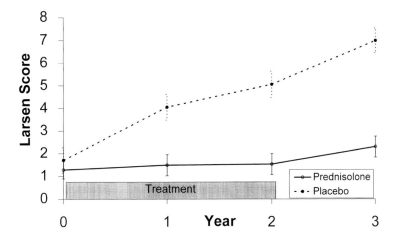

Figure 1b. Mean (95% CI) Larsen score after log transformation for 75 patients with radiographs at all time points. The difference between groups is significant at 1, 2 and 3 years.

Table 4. Proportion of hand radiographs which had no erosions in the ARC study [9, 10]

	Treatment group	
	Prednisolone	Placebo
At entry	27.8	28.2
After 2 years of treatment	34.7	59.0
After a further year of no treatment	39.2	66.5

In a study from the Netherlands (the COBRA study [11]), 76 test and 79 control patients received continuous sulphasalazine. The test subjects were also treated with methotrexate for 40 weeks and prednisolone for 28 weeks. The daily prednisolone dose was 60 mg in week 1, 40 mg in week 2, 25 mg in week 3, 20 mg in week 4, 15 mg in week 5, 10 mg in week 6, and 7.5 mg thereafter. Both methotrexate and prednisolone were discontinued gradually. The radiographic results are illustrated in Figure 2. Hand and feet radiographs were included in this study and were assessed using an erosion score devised for the study [11]. Erosive progression was prevented during the period of treatment with prednisolone and methotrexate in addition to sulphasalazine. In this study the benefits of the prednisolone seemed to persist for several weeks after treatment was discontinued, but erosive progression resumed between 56 and 80 weeks.

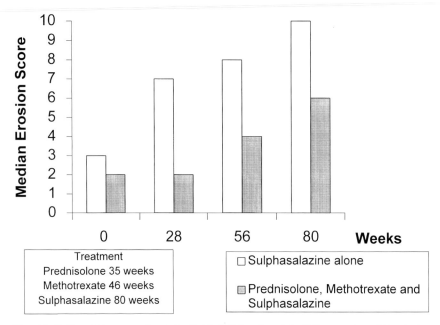

Figure 2. Radiographic progression in the Dutch Collaborative study [11] comparing sulphasalazine, methotrexate and prednisolone with sulphasalazine alone.

Implications of long-term glucocorticoid treatment response for disease pathology

An important observation made in several of these studies is that there was a dissociation between the response of different aspects of RA to glucocorticoid treatment. Compared to the placebo group, any increased suppression of the acute phase response had been lost by 3 months. Beneficial reduction in the symptoms of synovitis was evident in response to glucocortioids, but only for 6–9 months. In contrast, control of radiological progression was evident for the whole period of treatment.

This observation does not fit well with the traditional model of RA in which erosive change is a direct consequence of synovitis. Evidence is now accumulating that the process of synovitis is T-cell driven while that of cartilage and bone destruction may be more macrophage mediated [27]. Thus the causative link between synovitis and erosions is less convincing. Furthermore, in the ARC study, glucocorticoids did not alter the acute phase response (except possibly in the very early weeks), suggesting that it, too, is not necessarily related to synovitis or erosions in a causal way. A re-analysis of some of the data from the ARC study demonstrated [27a] that the correlation between the ongoing presence of synovitis and erosive progression in individual joints of the hand was weak (r = 0.248) and explained only 6% of the variance in measurements. These findings argue against there being a direct causal relationship between synovitis and erosions. Persistently observed synovitis in a joint was often not associated with x-ray progression at that joint and nearly half of those joints which did develop progressive damage had shown little evidence of clinical synovitis. A more appropriate model of RA, which can accommodate these observations and is similar to that advocated by Kirwan and Currey [28] is shown in Figure 3. This model is open to a variety of tests, such as finding out whether the histology of synovitis correlates with clinical progression; whether joint space narrowing and erosions are dissociated in clinical studies; whether other differential treatment effects can be demonstrated; and whether there are different risk factors and prognostic indicators for erosive and non-erosive disease. It will be of interest to observe the emergence of the data from studies addressing these issues.

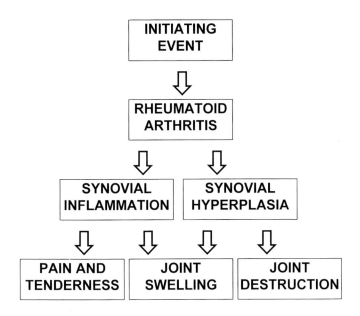

Figure 3. A model of rheumatoid arthritis consistent with the currently available data.

Logical treatment strategies for glucocorticoids in inflammatory arthritis

Although glucocorticoids cannot be recommended for all patients with RA, there are certain situations in which they may be the preferred treatment for symptom control. Owing to their relatively good safety profile glucocorticoids may be used during arthritic flare ups in pregnancy. Low dose prednisolone may be a preferable alternative to non-steroidal anti-inflammatory drugs in the elderly in order to avoid aggravation of renal or cardiac failure. The use of high dose glucocorticoids in systemic and vasculitic crises is widely practised [29] (see below). From the evidence of the MRC and ARC trials reviewed above, there is a case for using 7.5 mg prednisolone to treat some patients with RA in the early years of their disease (Tab. 5). Treating non-erosive patients more than 3 years after diagnosis will result in no benefit, as such patients are extremely unlikely to develop radiological change [30]. The published findings for radiological protection could reasonably be extrapolated into the fourth and fifth years of disease, but further extension of these findings would be difficult to justify without additional evidence of efficacy.

Table 5. Policy for selecting and treating patients with prednisolone 7.5 mg daily. Patients should have active inflammatory disease and all other treatment modalities should be used as clinically indicated

Erosion Status	Disease duration (years)		
	1–2	3–4	>4
Erosive	Treat for 2–4 years then stop	Probably treat for 2 years then stop	Do not treat as risk-benefit ratio is unknown
Non-erosive	Treat for 2–4 years then stop	Do not treat as probably will never be erosive	Do not treat as probably will never be erosive

Discontinuation of therapy should be by rapid tapering off. One suitable regimen is alternateday treatment for 2 weeks then every third day for 2 weeks, then stop [9, 10].

Adverse effects of glucocorticoid treatment

In the treatment of any disease which is not immediately fatal, the benefits must be weighed against the adverse effects that can be produced by the treatment. In studies of the frequency of adverse effects of glucocorticoids at low doses, it has been shown that weight gain, skin changes, hypertension, peptic ulceration and adrenal suppression are not increased [32, 33]. Although some studies have shown an adverse effect of glucocorticoids on bone loss even at small doses, the subject of osteoporosis is controversial. The evidence for glucocorticoid-induced osteoporosis cautions against routine use in premenopausal women [34]. There is, however, an independent risk of osteoporosis in RA. Patients on glucocorticoids tend to have more severe disease and as such are at greater risk of osteoporosis due to the disease itself and the associated functional disability. The improved function resulting from glucocorticoid treatment would reduce the rate of bone loss because of increased functional activity, which has a positive effect on bone density. Finally, even if low dose glucocorticoid treatment does cause increased bone loss in RA it is not entirely clear how this translates into clinically important fractures, even though there is evidence that fracture risk is partially related to the total cumulative steroid dose [34]. There is some evidence that supplementation with biphosphanates and/or hormone replacement therapy may retard bone loss with the potential to reduce the frequency of fractures [34, 35].

Information is beginning to accumulate that prolonged corticosteroid therapy may accelerate the development of atherosclerosis [36]. Lower limb atherosclerosis may occur in as many as 60% of corticosteroid-treated patients with RA. Several studies of mortality in RA and other connective tissue diseases have detected an increased cardiovascular mortality among sufferers, suggesting an approximate doubling in the death rate from ischemic heart disease. Although data on corticosteroid use in these studies are often incomplete, one study reported an excess of coronary artery deaths in a corticosteroid-treated group when compared with a noncorticosteroid-treated control group [19]. The evidence linking corticosteroid therapy with atherosclerosis falls far short of proof, but if true, even a small effect would have considerable clinical significance.

One reasonable approach allowing for bone and cardiovascular complications may be to avoid prescribing glucocorticoids in patients at high risk of serious adverse effects. These include: thin, frail, elderly women; patients with a history of serious cardiovascular disease (ischaemic heart disease, hypercholesterolaemia and hypertension) and those with poorly controlled diabetes.

High dose pulsed glucocorticoids in systemic RA or lupus nephritis and vasculitis

Pulse therapy involves the i.v. infusion of a large dose of corticosteroid (usually 1 g of methylprednisolone) over a short time, perhaps 30 min. A variety of regimens are used currently, but most entail a course of three pulses on alternate days, followed by a resting phase of around 6 weeks. This form of treatment was initiated in renal transplant recipients, but gradually spread to the treatment of other renal disorders, most notably lupus nephritis. The observation was made in such patients that synovial inflammation responded rapidly, and for prolonged periods, with i.v. therapy. Following anecdotal reports of benefit in RA, controlled studies were performed through the 1980s that suggested beneficial effects lasting 6–12 weeks from this regimen with relatively few side-effects [36]. These trials are small, however, and therefore limited in statistical power.

Methylprednisolone has been used in a number of studies to produce an early initial response in RA patients commencing second-line agents, thus effectively bridging the gap between initiation and response with these agents. A recent review [37] of the use of pulsed methylprednisolone stresses the impressive favourable risk : benefit ratio of this therapy with few or minor adverse effects. Most of the serious adverse effects: cardiovascular collapse, myocardial infarction, severe infection, have occurred in patients with compromised cardiovascular or immune systems as a result of their disease, or due to concomitant drug treatment. The minimal effective dose of methylprednisolone is uncertain at present. It has been reported that doses as low as 320 mg may be as effective as 1 g [38] although others [39] have concluded that using only 500 mg results in substantial loss of efficacy. If equivalent oral doses are as effective as i.v. treatment [40], this will allow pulsed treatment to become an outpatient procedure with reduced costs and less patient discomfort, although Choy et al. [41] found that intramuscular methylprednisolone was superior to equivalent oral doses in their study of corticosteroids and gold therapy.

In experimental models of vasculitis, such as serum sickness, circulating immune complexes activate platelets, deposit in blood vessel walls fixing complement and induce chemotaxis and phagocytosis by polymorphonuclear leukocytes with the release of enzymes that cause tissue damage. Aggregates of activated platelets form a nidus for blood coagulation and release thromboxane, which itself propagates further platelet activation, vasoconstriction and thrombus formation. In some vasculitides, such as Kawakaki's syndrome and Takayasu's disease, there is evidence of such a coagulopathy with hyperfibrinogenemia and hypofibrinolytic activity, which may result in luminal occluson [42]. Corticosteroids are widely used to treat systemic vasculities in RA, systemic lupus erythematosus (SLE) and other autoimmune diseases and are clearly powerful inhibitors of the inflammatory processes. However, corticosteroids may not inhibit subsequent organisation of the platelet and fibrin thrombus and induction of endothelial cell and smooth muscle cell proliferation. Thus, in spite of clinical and laboratory improvement after corticosteroid treatment, patients may go on to develop evidence of progressive ischemia, such as blue digits. Conn et al. [42] suggests that where there is no clinical evidence of active inflammation indicated by fever, myalgia, arthralgias or active skin lesions, and no laboratory evidence of inflammation such as elevation of the erythrocyte sedimentation rate (ESR), a more plausible management strategy would be the use of vasodilators and inhibitors of platelet activation. They postulate that corticosteroids fail to control the generation of platelet-dervied thromboxane, but it may be that this deficiency is often offset by the concomitant, widespread use of (platelet suppressing) NSAIDs.

Reports of complications following pulse corticosteroid therapy [36] have usually arisen in renal transplant patients (Tab. 6). Most important among these is sudden death, most probably arising as a result of ventricular dysrhythmia and consequent myocardial infarction. In three such cases, the i.v. bolus was administered rapidly (in one case over only 20 s) and all were taking furosemide (frusemide), which may have induced hypokalemia. It has been suggested that increasing the infusion time to at least 30 min might prevent such events. Nevertheless, the incidence of such sudden death appears to be extremely low, given that well over 10 000 renal transplant patients are likely to have been treated with pulse corticosteroids. Other reported complications

Table 6. Adverse effects of systemic corticosteroid therapy.

Metabolic	Obesity
	Glucose/protein metabolism
	Electrolyte imbalance
	Enzyme induction
Predisposition to infection	
Musculoskeletal	Myopathy
	Osteoporosis
	Osteonecrosis
	Tendon rupture
	Corticosteroid withdrawal syndrome
Gastrointestinal	Peptic ulcer disease
	Pancreatitis
Ophthalmic	Cataract
	Glaucoma
Central nervous system	Psychosis
	Depression
	Benign intracranial hypertension
Dermatologic	Acne
	Striae
	Alopecia
	Bruising
	Skin atrophy
Growth retardation	
Hypothalamic-pituitary-adrenal axis suppression	

include transient arthralgias and synovitis, hyperglycemia, pancreatitis, gastrointestinal bleeding, visual disturbance and acute psychosis.

Fatal infections have also been reported. However, these are rare, and have occurred in transplant patients on daily doses of azathioprine, often following continued, long-term use of 1 g pulses. *In vitro* studies indicate, however, that methylprednisolone pulses fail to reduce bacterial phagocytosis or killing by human neutrophils.

Corticosteroids in polymalgia rheumatica and temporal arteritis

The signs and symptoms of polymyalgia rheumatica (PMR) and temporal arteritis (TA) overlap and can often be confused, but both are treated with corticosteroids. No controlled trials have been conducted which allow adequate definition of the best treatment regimen, but three cohorts of patients and their use of corticosteroids have been reported in the literature [43–45]. Although there are some differences, the overall pattern suggests the need to treat PMR initially with about 15 mg prednisolone daily, reducing slowly over 18–24

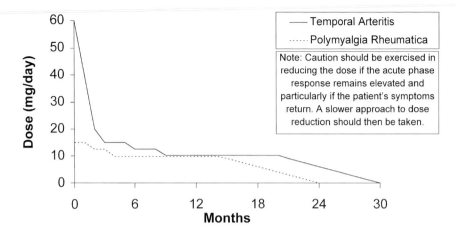

Figure 4. Typical dose regimens for treating polymyalgia rheumatica and temporal arteritis with prednisolone.

months. About twice that dose of corticosteroids will be required to treat coex-
isting or separate TA and for perhaps 6 months longer. Figure 4 illustrates
appropriate dose levels, although caution should be exercised in reducing the
dose if the acute phase response remains elevated and particularly if the
patient's symptoms return. A slower approach to dose reduction should then be
taken. Clinical experience suggests that some patients will be unable to stop
glucocorticoids completely.

All series reported a few complications, including some patients with PMR
who developed more definite TA while on treatment. The main pitfalls seem to
be the use of too high a dose of corticosteroids initially, with a too rapid reduction in treatment thereafter [46]. The cause of symptoms in PMR, particulaly
morning stiffness, is unknown, and does not seem to be related to clinical signs
of inflammation. It will be intriguing to discover why glucocorticoids are so
effective in this condition.

References

1 Hench PS, Kendall EC, Slocumb CH, Polley HF (1949) Effects of a hormone of the adrenal cortex (17-hydroxy-11 dehydrocorticosterone: compound E) and of pituitary adrenocorticotrophic
  hormone on rheumatoid arthritis. Preliminary report. *Proceedings Staff Meetings Mayo Clinic* 24:
  181–197
2 Kirwan JRSilman AJ (1987) Epidemiological, social and environmental aspects of rheumatoid
  arthritis and osteoarthritis. *Bailliere Clin Rheumatol* 1: 467–489
3 Kirwan JR, South West Regional Advisory Committee for Rheumatology (1994) The effect of
  National Health Service reforms on outpatient rheumatology workload. *Brit J Rheumatol* 33:
  1181–1183
4 Pincus T (1988) Rheumatoid arthritis: disappointing long-term outcomes despite successful short
  term-clinical trials. *J Clin Epidemiol* 41: 1037–1041

5 Scott DL, Spector TD, Pullar T, McConkey B (1989) What should we hope to achieve when treating rheumatoid arthritis? *Ann Rheum Dis* 48: 256–261

6 Weisman MH (1993) Should steroids be used in the management of rheumatoid arthritis? *Rheum Dis Clin N Amer* 19: 189–199

7 Harris EDJr, Emkey RD, Nicholas JE, Newberg A (1983) Low dose prednisolone therapy in rheumatoid arthritis. A double blind study. *J Rheum* 10: 713–721

8 Weiss MM (1989) Corticosteroids in rheumatoid arthritis. *Semin Arthr Rheum* 19(1): 9–21

9 Kirwan JR, Byron M, Dieppe P, Eastmond C, Halsey J, Hickling P, Hollingworth P, Jacoby R, Kirk A, Moran C et al (1995) The effect of glucocorticoids on joint destruction in rheumatoid arthritis. *NEJM* 333: 3: 142–146

10 Hickling P, Jacoby RK, Kirwan JR, The Arthritis, Rheumatism Council Low-Dose Glucocorticoid Study Group (1998) Joint destruction after glucocorticoids are withdrawn in early rheumatoid arthritis. *Brit J Rheumatol* 37: 930–936

11 Boers M, Verhoeven AC, Markusse HM, van de Laar M, Westhovens R, van Denderen J, van Zeben D, Dijkmans B, Peeters A, Jacobs P (1997) Randomised comparison of combined step down prednisolone, methotrexate and sulphasalazine with sulphasalazine alone in early rheumatoid arthritis. *Lancet* 350: 309–318

12 Saag KG, Criswell LA, Sems KM, Nettleman MD, Kolluri S (1996) Low-dose corticosteroids in rheumatoid arthritis. A meta-analysisof their moderate-term effectiveness. *Arthritis Rheumatism* 39: 1818–1825

13 Panayi GS, Heberden Oration (1993) The pathogenesis of rheumatoid arthritis: From molecules to the whole patient. *Brit J Rheumatol* 32: 533–536

14 Chikanza IC, Petrou P, Kingsley G, Chrousos G, Panayi GS (1992) Defective hypothalamic response to immune and inflammatory stimuli in patients with rheumatoid arthritis. *Arthritis Rheumatism* 35: 1281–1288

15 Joint Committee of the Medical Research Council, Nuffield Foundation (1954) A comparison of cortisone and aspirin in the treatment of early cases of rheumatoid arthritis. *Brit Med J* 29: 1223–1227

16 Empire Rheumatism Council (1955) Multi-centre controlled trial comparing cortisone acetate and acetyl salicylic acid in the long-term treatment of rheumatoid arthritis. *Ann Rheum Dis* 14: 353–367

17 Joint Committee of the Medical Research Council, Nuffield Foundation (1959) A comparison of prednisolone with aspirin or other analgesics in the treatment of rheumatoid arthritis. *Ann Rheum Dis* 18: 173–187

18 Joint Committee of the Medical Research Council, Nuffield Foundation (1960) A comparison of prednisolone with aspirin or other analgesics in the treatment of rheumatoid arthritis. *Ann Rheum Dis* 19: 331–337

19 West HF (1967) Rheumatoid arthritis. The relevance of clinical knowledge to research activities. *Abstracts World Medicine* 41: 401–417

20 Masi AT (1983) Low dose glucocorticoid therapy in rheumatoid arthritis. *J Rheumatol* 10: 675–678

21 Berntsen CA, Freyberg RH (1961) Rheumatoid patients after five or more years of glucocorticoid treatment: A comparative analysis of 183 cases. *Ann Intern Med* 54: 938–953

22 Leibling MR, Leib E, McLaughlin K (1981) Pulse methyl-prednisolone in rheumatoid arthritis. *Ann Intern Med* 4: 21–26

23 Harris EDJr Emkey RD, Nichols JE, Newberg A (1983) Low dose prednisolone therapy in rheumatoid arthritis: A double blind study. *J Rheumatol* 10: 713–721

24 Million R, Poole P, Kellgren JH, Joyson J (1984) Long-term study of management of rheumatoid arthritis. *Lancet* 1: 812–816

25 Hansen TM, Kryger P, Elling H, Haar D, Kreutzfeldt M, Ingeman-Nielsen MW, Olsson AT, Pedersen C, Rahbek A, Tvede N, Winge J (1990) Double blind placebo controlled trial of pulse treatment with methylprednisolone combined with disease modifying drugs in rheumatoid arthritis. *BMJ* 301: 268–270

26 Byron MA, Kirwan JR (1986) Corticosteroids in rheumatoid arthritis: Is a trial of their 'disease modifying' potential feasible? *Ann Rheum Dis* 46: 171–173

27 Bresnihan B, Mulherin D, FitzGerald O (1995) Synovial pathology and articular erosions in rheumatoid arthritis. *Rheumatology in Europe* 24 (Suppl 2): 158–160

27a Kirwan JR (1997) The relationship between synovitis and erosions in rheumatoid arthritis. *Brit J Rheumatol* 36: 225–228

28 Kirwan JR, Currey HLF (1983) Rheumatoid arthritis: disease modifying anti-rheumatoid drugs. *Clin Rheum Dis* 9: 581–599
29 George E, Kirwan JR (1990) Glucocorticoid therapy in rheumatoid arthritis. *Bailliere Clin Rheum* 4: 621–647
30 Brook A, Corbett M (1977) Radiographic change in early rheumatoid disease. *Ann Rheumat Dis* 36: 71–73
31 Larsen A, Dale K, Eek M (1977) Radiographic evaluation of rheumatoid arthritis and related conditions by standard reference films. *Acta Radiologica* 18: 481–491
32 Caldwell JR, Furst DE (1991) The efficacy and safety of low-dose cortiosteroids for rheumatoid arthritis. *Sem Arthr Rheum* 21; 1: 1–11
33 Sambrook PN, Eisman JA, Ygates MG Pocock NA, Ebgrl S, Champion GD (1986) Osteoporosis in rheumatoid arthritis: safety of low dose corticosteroids. *Ann Rheumat Dis* 45: 950–953
34 Hall GM, Spector TD, Griffin AJ, Jawad ASM, Hall ML, Doyle DV (1993) The effect of rheumatoid arthritis and steroid therapy on bone density in postmenopausal women. *Arthritis Rheum* 36: 11: 1510–1516
35 Adachi JD, Cranney A, Goldsmith CH et al (1994) Intermittent cyclic therapy with etidronate in the prevention of glucocorticoid induced bone loss. *J Rheumatol* 21; 10: 1922–1926
36 Cooper C, Kirwan JR (1990) The risk of local and systemic corticosteroid administration. *Bailliere Clin Rheumatol* 4: 305–332
37 Weusten BLAM, Jacobs JWG, Bijlsma JWJ (1993) Corticosteroid pulse therapy in active rheumatoid arthritis. *Semin Arthritis Rheum* 23: 183–192
38 Radia M, Furst DE (1988) Comparison of three pulse methylprednisolone regimens in the treatment of rheumatoid arthritis. *J Rheumatol* 15: 242–256
39 Shipley ME, Bacon PA, Berry H, Hazleman BL, Sturrock RD, Swinson DR, Williams IA (1988) Pulsed methylprednisolone in active early rheumatoid disease. A dose ranging study. *Brit J Rheumatol* 27: 211–214
40 Needs CJ, Smith M, Boutagy J et al (1988) Comaprison of methylprednisolone (1 gram IV) with prednisolone (1 gram orally) in rheuamtoid arthritis: a pharmokinetic and clinical study. *J Rheumatol* 15: 224–228
41 Choy EHS, Kingsley G, Corkhill MM, Panayi GS (1993) Intramuscular methylprednisolone is superior to pulse oral methylprednisolone during the induction phase of chrysotherapy. *Brit J Rheumatol* 32: 734–739
42 Conn D, Tomkins RB, Nichols WL (1988) Glucocorticoids in the management of vasculitis-a double edged sword? *J Rheumatol* 15(5): 1181–1183
43 Salvarini C, Macchioni PL, Tartoni PL, Rossi F, Baricchi R, Castri C, Ciaravallot IF, Portioli I (1987) Polymyalgia rheumatica and giant cell arteritis: a 5-year rpidemiologic and clinical study in Reggio Emilia, Italy. *Clin Exp Rheumatol* 5: 205–215
44 Delecoeuillerie G, Joly P, de Lara AC, Paolaggi JB (1988) Polymyalgia rheumatica and temporal arteritis: a retrospective analysis of prognostic features and different corticosteroid regimens (11 year survey of 210 patients). *Ann Rheum Dis* 47: 733–739
45 Lundberg I, Hedfors E (1990) Restricted dose and duration of corticosteroid treatment in patients with polymyalgia rheumatica and temporal arteritis. *J Rheumatol* 17: 1340–1345
46 Kirwan JR (1990) Treatment of polymyalgia rheumatica. *Brit J Rheumatol* 29: 316

Glucocorticoids
ed. by N.J. Goulding and R.J. Flower
© 2001 Birkhäuser Verlag/Switzerland

Glucocorticoids in the control of inflammatory bowel disease

Filip J. Baert and Paul R. Rutgeerts

Department of Gastroenterology at the University Hospital Gasthuisberg, Leuven, Belgium

Introduction

Inflammatory bowel disease (IBD) constitutes a group of chronic idiopathic inflammatory bowel conditions commonly subdivided into Crohn's disease (CD), involving commonly the small bowel and or colon, and ulcerative colitis (UC), a condition confined to parts of or the entire large bowel (colon). About 5 to 10 per 100 000 inhabitants in Western countries are affected, with a peak incidence of onset of disease in their twenties causing a considerable burden, with usually need for chronic medications and in about 30–50% of patients need for surgery.

Although the exact nature and cause of these conditions remain obscure considerable progress has been made in recent years, not only in the treatment, but also in unraveling the pathogenesis [1]. The current consensus is that the inflammation is caused when cytokines are triggered by exposure of the intestinal mucosa to common antigens in the faecal stream. Some individuals are genetically predisposed, but other environmental factors, for example, smoking, exposures to viruses etc. may be involved. The inflammation seems to be orchestrated by T-helper-1 lymphocytes producing a variety of pro-inflammatory cytokines (TNF-α, IFN-γ, IL-1, etc.). In turn these cytokines interact in a very complex way with an impressive array of immunocompetent cells (e.g., monocytes, lymphocytes but also eosinophils, dendritic cells, endothelial cells and epithelial cells) and molecules (e.g., adhesion molecules, metalloproteinases, transcription factors, heat shock proteins, oxygen radicals, arachidonic acid metabolites, etc...).

Although glucocorticoids have very broad and non specific effects in this cascade of inflammatory mediators they are still the mainstay of therapy in IBD. In trying to minimize side-effects recent developments focus on avoiding the use and shortening the duration of classic steroid therapy. This can be realized by using immunomodulatory (so-called steroid sparing) agents, or by using new, very specific, genetically engineered monoclonal antibody approaches (e.g., anti TNF antibodies). Another considerable progress is the development of new synthetic agents with high topical activity and low systemic bio-availability thereby greatly reducing side-effects. Finally, surgical alternatives in IBD patients, both CD and UC, with disease locations amenable to resections, may be more appropriate.

Actions and pharmacokinetics of glucorticoids in IBD

Classic glucocorticoids (e.g., prednisone of methylprednisolone), whether used orally, intravenously or as an enema, will induce a mix of topical and systemic activities in IBD patients. GCS have a high oral bio-availability, relatively high systemic absorption combined with a low hepatic first-pass effect. Therefore, as in other conditions, steroid therapy will trigger the glucocorticoid receptor (GCS-R) throughout the body and will suppress the hypothalamic pituitary adrenal axis. This explains the scala of the observed effects and side-effects.

This GCS-R influences, through an intracellular signal transduction pathway, the transcription, translation and breakdown of a wide variety of key players in the inflammatory cascade inducing clinically very important functional changes.

The proposed major anti-inflammatory immunosuppressive mechanisms of GCS have been extended over time as new mediators were discovered. Today the central role of cytokines in cellular cross -talk, activation and recruitment is in focus. The modulation of cytokine expression through different genomic mechanisms is one of the key mechanisms of action. It is generally accepted that GCS inhibit cytokine production. In reality the effects may be much more complex. GCS effects may be tissue specific and dependent on the phase (initial *versus* extensive) of inflammation. Moreover the effect will depend on the type of cell and type of stimulus. Some examples of *in vitro effects* are given in Table 1. Finally, very little is known what GCS do *in vivo* to the inflamed bowel mucosa [2, 3].

Because the GCS-R are not organ specific, it has not been possible to develop new steroids with different actions at the receptor level. However by mod-

Table 1. Examples of *in vitro* modulation of cytokine expression by GCS and subsequent functional changes

Cytokine	Cell	Stimulus	Effect	Functional changes
IL1β	Monocytes	LPS	↓	↓ Antigen presentation, Lymphocyte proliferation
TNF-α	Lymphocytes		↓	and apoptosis
Il-8	Monocytes	LPS, TNF, IL1β	↓	↓ Recruitment of inflammatory cells
IL-10	Lymphocytes	LPS	↓	
TGF-β	Lymphocytes	mitogens	↑↓	↓ Wound healing
PDGF	Macrophages	IFN γ	↑↓	and fibrosis

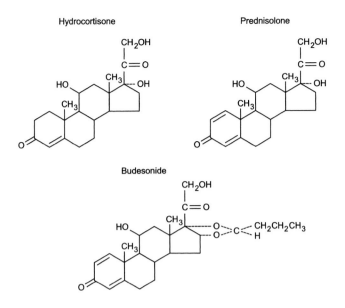

Figure 1. The structure of the main compounds with steroid actions.

ifying the structure of the substituents on the steroid skeleton (see Fig. 1) it has been possible to influence the specific affinity for the GCS-R, the absorption and dwell time at the site of application and most importantly the rate of first pass inactivation by the liver. In theory, these properties should allow maximal topical action and considerably reduce steroid levels in the systemic circulation. The new semi-synthetic corticosteroids (toxicortol pivalate, beclomethasone dipropionate, and budesonide), all carry a lipophilic 17α- and/or 16α- substitution, resulting in a much higher affinity for the GCS-R and undergoing extensive first-pass hepatic inactivation. Most clinical experience in IBD with these new formulations is with budesonide. (Tab. 2) Budesonide

Table 2. Pharmacological properties of the major glucocorticosteroids used in IBD[*]

Compound	Antiinflam-matory effect	Mineralo-corticoid effect	Bio-availability oral (%)	Plasma t1/2 (min)	Biological t1/2 (hours)	Receptor affinity
Hydrocortisone	1	++	50–60	90	8–12	1
Prednisone	4	+	80	200	12–36	13
Methyl-prednisolone	5	–	65–70	180	12–36	13
Budesonide	200	–	10–15	90–270	?	200

[*] Adapted from D'Haens GR, Rutgeerts PJ (1996) How should corticosteroids be used in inflammatory bowel disease? *Clin Immunother* 5: 334–340

is commercially available in an enema form (Entocort, Astra Pharmaceuticals) for distal or left-sided colitis, and in an oral, slow release galenic form (Budenofalk, Dr Falk Pharma), and a controlled ileal release capsule (Entocort, Astra Pharmaceuticals) which reaches the terminal ileum and right colon. After oral or rectal administration budesonide induces very high steroid topical activity in the ileum and left colon, it is then absorbed and drained through the intestinal circulation to the liver were it is for the most part inactivated leaving little steroid activity in the systemic circulation (Fig. 2). The key pharmacological and pharmacokinetic properties of the principal compounds with steroid actions are given in Table 2. The oral bio-availability of classic steroids ranges from 50–80%. Although the plasma half-life is limited to only a few hours, the biological half-life extends up to 12 to 36 h. For budesonide the high receptor affinity and low oral bio-availability explains the beneficial efficacy/toxicity ratio [4].

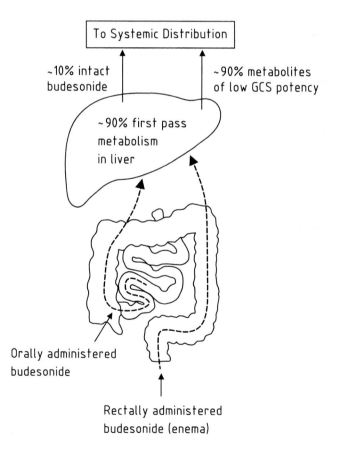

Figure 2. Budesonide (administered orally or as enema) undergoes extensive first pass effect in the liver.

General recommendations and practical guidelines for the use of glucocorticoids in IBD

Systemic glucorticoids are still the single most effective commonly available drugs in the treatment of IBD. However their use should be restricted to moderately to severely ill patients, usually with systemic symptoms, e.g., weight loss, fever, anorexia, fatigue, extra intestinal manifestations (arthritis, eye or skin manifestations).

When glucocorticosteroids are initiated the usual starting dose should be sufficiently high. Standard 40 mg of prednisone (or equivalent 32 mg of methylprednisolone) as a single oral morning dose is employed for at least 2 weeks. Enteric infections as reasons for flares should be excluded by negative coproculture and stool exams for parasites and *Clostridium difficile* toxin. In Crohn's patients with an inflammatory mass or abscess broad spectrum antibiotics including coverage for anaerobes should be started concomitantly. In patients responding this dose is usually continued for 2–4 weeks or until a significant clinical improvement has been achieved. This dose can be tapered off by 4 mg per week to 16 mg, and then by usually 4 mg every 2 weeks thereafter. As steroids do not have a role in preventing relapse of disease both in CD and UC an attempt to stop the steroids completely is always warranted. Therefore tapering off of steroids should be accompanied by starting or optimizing a maintenance drug (see below). Most patients, especially after long-term therapy, will experience non specific symptoms such as fatigue, myalgia and sore joints when stopping therapy. It is important to realize that these symptoms are likely to be steroid induced and not a manifestation of the disease. They should therefore never be a reason to not discontinue steroid therapy.

In patients truly refractory to glucocorticoids alternative therapies, including surgery, should be considered and steroids may be stopped suddenly or tapered off faster. Alternatively patients with insufficient response to oral steroids can be admitted for intravenous therapy and enteral or parenteral nutrition. Intravenous dosing of 40 to 60 mg of methylprednisolone or equiv-

Table 3. Strategies to minimize steroid related side-effects.

---

1. Always consider alternative therapies (surgery, antibiotics, enteral nutrition)

2. Substitute by or switch to budesonide if possible

3. Optimize maintenance therapy and dosages (5-ASA 3–4 g/d, azathioprine 2–2.5 mg/kg/d)

4. Look for potential external causes for flares (infections, compliance, smoking, NSAIDs)

5. Correct dosing and tapering regimen

6. Discontinue in true refractory patients

7. Taper steroids always completely (no role in maintenance)

8. Address patients concerns regarding side-effects and prevent where possible

---

(see text)

alent is recommended. Higher dosing is probably of marginal benefit and may increase toxicity considerably. Although a single daily injection is most logical from a pharmacodynamic point of view, continuous IV infusion is commonly used.

Budesonide is the single most used "topical acting" steroid. In its oral form used for delivery to the ileocaecal region the recommended dosage regimen is three tablets of 3 mg. Both single morning dosing and three times per day dosing have been recommended. Marginal dose responses can be expected above 9 mg daily. Generally, clinical remission is obtained after 4 to 8 weeks, thereafter slow and gradual tapering off is recommended. In steroid dependent patients an attempt can be made to switch from prednisone to budesonide with overall success in 50 to 70% of patients [5].

Ulcerative colitis

Proctitis and left-sided colitis

Mild to moderate disease is usually amenable to aminosalicylate therapy. Topical glucocorticoids such as hydrocortisone foam (for proctitis) or hydrocortisone or budesonide enemas (for proctosigmoiditis) can be employed alone or in combination with oral aminosalicylates to treat acute disease. Thereafter clinical remission should be maintained with either oral or topical aminosalicylates.

Pancolitis

In patients with more extensive colitis especially with moderate or severe symptoms systemic GCS are the first choice of therapy. Methylprednisolone at an oral dosage of 32 mg (or equivalent) should be started until all symptoms abate. Tapering off should then be initiated at a rate corresponding to the length of the time required to induce remission. In all cases an attempt should be made to discontinue the steroids completely. In most cases patients will be maintained on aminosalicylates or azathioprine/6- mercaptopurine [6].

In patients with worsening symptoms or refractory disease to a high oral dose of steroids admission for in-hospital intravenous treatment is indicated. Parenteral steroids can be given as a continuous infusion of 40 mg of methylprednisolone or as 300–400 mg of hydrocortisone or an equivalent. If symptoms persist after 7–10 days of this regimen, colectomy should be seriously considered. Alternatively, a continuous infusion of cyclosporin can be effective, at least initially, in delaying acute surgical intervention. However long-term beneficial effects of cyclosporin are more controversial [7, 8].

Crohn's disease

Classic systemic steroid therapy

Two large scale studies have demonstrated the effect of oral GCS for active Crohn's disease. In the National Cooperative Crohn's disease study (NCCDS) remission was achieved with prednisone 0.25 to 0.75 mg/kg/d in 60% of patients *versus* 30% in the placebo group [9]. In the European Cooperative Crohn's disease study (ECCDS), 80% of patients had achieved remission after 100 days of methylprednisolone *versus* 15% with placebo [10]. There was no additional benefit from sulfasalazine in either of these trials. Sometimes a combination of broad spectrum antibiotics may be an alternative for steroid in the treatment of an acute flare up [11].

Munckholm et al., in a very elegant study, looked at the immediate (<30 days) and prolonged (30 days after stopping) outcome of a first course of GCS therapy in Crohn's disease as a single agent. Complete remission was obtained in 48% of patients, partial remission in 32% and no response in 20% within 30 days of treatment. Prolonged steroid response was noted in 44%, steroid dependency in 36% and steroid resistance in 20% of patients. The observed responses were irrespective of disease location, age, sex or clinical symptoms [12].

When oral GCS fail it is generally accepted that intravenous GCS may be of additional benefit along with general supportive measures such as bowel rest, enteral or parenteral nutrition, and broad spectrum antibiotics.

As in ulcerative colitis there is no role for steroids in maintenance therapy. Several studies have shown continuous therapy with a low dose of steroids does not prevent flare ups of the disease. Most patients with refractory disease or recurrent flare ups with need for steroid therapy will need additional maintenance therapy with immunomodulating agents. First choice here is azathioprine or 6-mercaptopurine. The effects of azathioprine are more then just steroid sparing. Compared to steroids alone, patients on the combination azathioprine and prednisone will achieve a complete remission more rapidly and more frequently (with lower doses of prednisone) [13].

Switching from systemic steroids when tapering off, to budesonide (see below) may be a valuable alternative to avoid side-effects.

Topical acting agent: budesonide

For patients with disease located in the terminal ileum and or ascending colon topical GCS have been developed. Most clinical experience has been gathered with budesonide. The controlled ileal formulations (CIR) treatment contain acid-stable microgranules of budesonide that dissolve at a pH above 5.5 to 6.4. This explains why these "enteric" coated forms of budesonide act topically in the ileocaecal region. Although budesonide CIR cause a dose related reduction in basal ACTH stimulated plasma cortisol levels, clinically important corticosteroid related side-effects are limited [4].

Several trials have demonstrated clear clinical benefit almost equal to systemic steroids at an optimal dosage of 9 mg/day. In an 8-week, placebo controlled trial for active Crohn's disease remission occurred in 51% of patients compared to 20% of placebo patients (p < 0.001) [14]. Two large trials compared budesonide to systemic steroids. After 8 to 10 weeks of budesonide treatment 53 to 60% of patients reached a complete remission compared to 60 to 63% in the prednisone group (NS). But the mean reductions in the Crohn's disease activity index are greater in the prednisone group (p = 0.001). Corticosteroid related side-effects were significantly less common in the budesonide group [15, 16]. The general conclusion is that a single dose of 9 mg budesonide CIR is as promptly effective as prednisolone and represents a safer therapeutic approach with fewer side-effects. Unfortunately as for classic GCS there seems to be no role for budesonide in maintenance therapy.

Strategies to minimize side-effects

Although very effective, the use of steroids is certainly not popular among patients. Therefore, is seems essential to anticipate problems by discussing the use of these agents with your patient before starting. Compliance and patient's satisfaction will increase by making correct assessments with your patient about long-term treatment aims and duration of therapy. Possible alternatives and concerns about toxicity, including previous individual experiences should be addressed.

Alternative therapies, for example, increasing mesalazine (5-ASA) doses to 3 to 4 g, combination of antibiotics, budesonide, enteral nutrition (especially in pediatric patients) and surgery should always be considered before starting steroids. The recurrent need for steroid therapy for flare-ups of the disease implies an insufficient maintenance therapy. Optimal maintenance regimens include 3 to 4 g of 5-ASA or 2 to 2.5 mg/kg of azathioprine. Because of the slow actions of the antimetabolites (azathioprine or mercaptopurine) they should be started early enough at a sufficient dose and for at least 3 to 6 months before they are considered ineffective. Alternatively an intravenous loading dose of azathioprine has been proposed [17]. About 20% of patients will show no response to steroids. In these patients therapy can be stopped abruptly in time to prevent Addison-like manifestations.

In terms of specific side-effects gastro-intestinal intolerance is usually avoided by taking the pills with meals. Only rarely antacids may be needed. In contrast to what is widely believed steroid therapy will not induce peptic ulcer disease. However the combination of non steroidal anti inflammatory drugs (NSAIDs) with steroids can be even more toxic for the gastric mucosa. In general, the use of aspirin and NSAIDs are contra indicated in IBD patients as they may worsen disease activity and symptoms. In the prevention of steroid related osteoporosis several drugs can be used. Apart from oral bifosfonates most drugs will exert only marginal effects once osteoporosis is induced. Although most clinicians start to worry about the osteoporosis when prescribing steroids for longer periods, several studies have shown that bone loss is most pronounced early in the steroid course. Therefore prevention early on may be warranted. We recommend among other measures to promote physical activity, to stop smoking and prescribe calcium supplements when steroids are initiated. Osteonecrosis (aseptic necrosis) affecting most often the femoral head or knees in about 1% of steroid treated patients, and corticoid induced myopathy do not depend on either dosage or duration of treatment.

Acne and acne like skin changes can be very disturbing in this young group of patients. In patients prone to these manifestations acne can be almost completely prevented with oral tetracycline preparations.

Emotional disturbances, mood swings and sleeplessness are common and more difficult to handle but should be addressed appropriately. Patients should be reassured that these side-effects are drug induced and reversible upon discontinuation. Real psychiatric syndromes like psychotic events and depression are rare but can occur especially with higher dosages. It is crucial to detect these symptoms early on as prompt actions should be taken. The occurrence of these side-effects should be contra indications for further steroid use.

In the pediatric age group steroid induced growth retardation is a special concern. Although not treating active inflammation may inhibit normal growth, every effort should be undertaken to minimize steroid use in these patients. As in the adult age group a more aggressive approach, using immunomodulating agents, is advocated in the refractory pediatric patients. Alternate day use of steroids is popular and enteral nutrition is a valid alternative for steroid therapy [18].

Conclusions

Although classic corticosteroids are still very effective in the control of inflammatory bowel diseases their use has gradually declined in the last decade. For mild to moderate disease safer alternatives are used including mesalamine in higher dosages, antibiotic regimens, budesonide. In severe or refractory disease better surgical techniques (ileo anal pouch anatomosis, stricturoplasties) and a more aggressive medical approach using immunomodulators (azathioprine, methotrexate, cyclosporin) obviate or limit their use. Furthermore their should be no longer a role for steroids (systemic or topical) as maintenance therapy in inflammatory bowel diseases.

Undoubtedly a better understanding of these conditions leading to rationally designed new agents with molecular biologic techniques, e.g., anti TNF and more to come, will further limit the use of steroids.

Finally, when prescribing steroids, physicians should address patient's concerns and try to prevent or treat side-effects wherever possible.

References

1 Fiocchi C (1998) Inflammatory bowel disease: etiology and pathogenesis. *Gastroenterology* 115: 182–205
2 Wilckens T, De Rijk R (1997) Glucocorticoids and immune function: unknown dimensions and new frontiers. *Immunol Today* 18: 418–423
3 Bratts R, Linden M (1996) Cytokine modulation by glucocorticoids: mechanisms and actions in cellular studies. *Aliment Pharmacol Ther* 10: 81–90
4 Jewell D, Rutgeerts P (eds) (1993) Reviewing steroids in the treatment of IBD. *Res Clin Forum* 15
5 Cortot A, Colombel JF, Rutgeerts P, Lauritsen K, Malchow H, Hamling J, Winter T, Pallant D, Petterson E (1999) Budesonide controlled ileal release capsules in prednisone dependent patient's with Crohn's disease. *Gastroenterology* 116:G3014
6 Hanauer S, Baert F (1995) The management of ulcerative colitis. *Annu Rev Med* 46: 497–505
7 Lichtiger S, Present D, Kornbluth A (1994) Cyclosporin in severe ulcerative colitis refractroy to steroid therapy. *N Engl J Med* 330: 1841–1850
8 Baert F, Hanauer S (1994) Cyclosporin in severe steroid resistant ulcerative colitis: long term results of therapy. *Gastroenterology* 106:A648
9 Summers RW, Switz DM, Sessions JT (1979) The national cooperative Crohn's idsease study: resuls of drug treatment. *Gastroenterology* 77: 847–869
10 Malchow Ewe K, Brandes JW (1984) European cooperative Crohn's disease study (ECCDS) results of drug treatment. *Gastroenterology* 86: 249–266
11 Prantera C, Zannoni F, Scribano ML, Berto E, Andreoli A, Kohn A, Luzi C (1996) An antibiotic regimen for the treatment of active Crohn's disease: a randomised controlled clinical trial of metronidazol and ciprofloxacin. *Amer J Gastroenterol* 91: 328–332
12 Munckholm P, Langholz E, Davidsen M, Binder V (1994) Frequency of glucocorticoid resistance and dependency in Crohn's disease. *Gut* 35: 360–362
13 Ewe K, Press AG, Singe CC, Stufler M, Ueberschaer B, Hommel G, Meyer zum Buschenfelde KH (1993) Azathioprine combined with prednisolone or monotherapy with prednisolone in active Crohn's disease. *Gastroenterology* 105: 367–372
14 Greenberg GR, Feagan BG, Martin F, Sutherlanbd LR, Thomson ABR, Williams CN, Nilsson LG, Persson T (1994) Oral budesoinde for active Crohn's disease. *N Engl J Med* 331: 836–841
15 Rutgeerts P, Löfberg R, Malchow H, Lmaers C, Olaison G, Jewell D, Danielsson A, Goebell H, Thomson OO, Lorenz Meyer H et al (1994) A comparison of budesonide with prednisolone for active Crohn's disease. *N Engl J Med* 331: 842–845
16 Campieri M, Ferguson A, Doe W, Persson T, L-GNilsson (1997) Oral budesonide is as effective as oral prednisolone in active Crohn's disease. *Gut* 41: 209–214
17 Sandborn WJ, Van Os EC, Zins BJ (1995) An intravenous loading dose of azathioprine decreases time to response in patients with Crohn's disease. *Gastroenterology* 109: 1808–1817
18 Wilschanski M, Sherman P, Pencharz P, Davis L, Corey M, Griffiths A (1996) Supplementary enteral nutrition maintains remission in paediatric Crohn's disease. *Gut* 38: 543–548

Subject index